The Mary Kay Guide to Beauty

The Mary Kay Guide to Beauty

Discovering Your Special Look

The Beauty Experts
at Mary Kay Cosmetics

▲ Addison-Wesley

Reading, Massachusetts Menlo Park, California
London Amsterdam Don Mills, Ontario Sydney

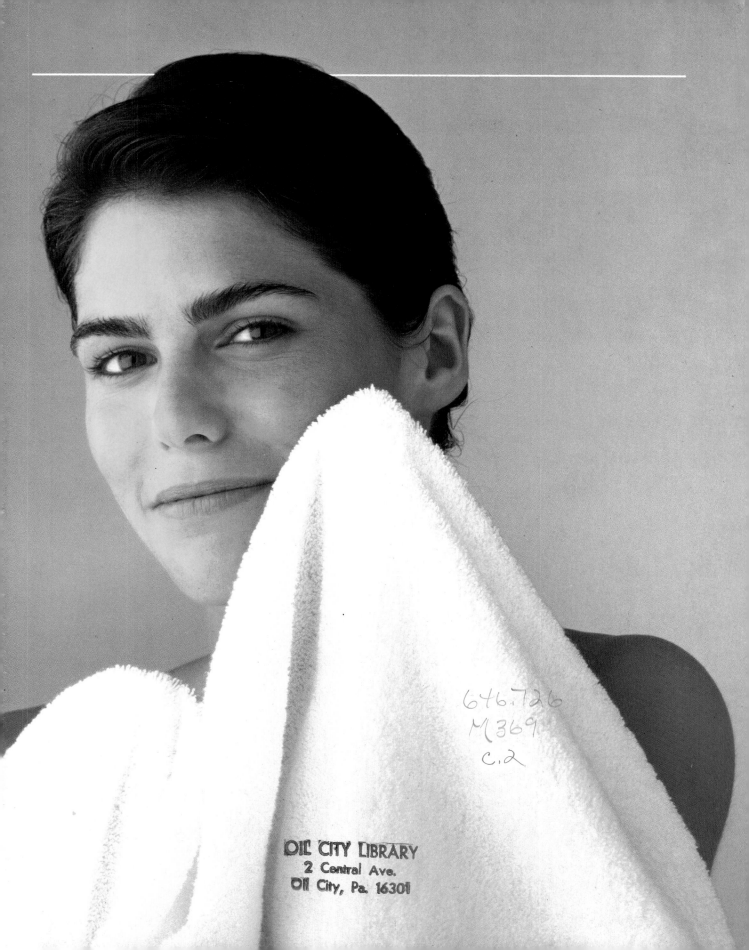

Library of Congress Cataloging in Publication Data
Main entry under title:

The Mary Kay guide to beauty

   1. Beauty, Personal.   2. Cosmetics.   I. Ash, Mary Kay.
   II. Mary Kay Cosmetics.

RA778.M374   1983   646.7'042   83-12235
ISBN 0-201-13990-1

ABCDEFGHIJ-KR-86543
First printing, August 1983

Writing	Susan Duff Elaine Raffel
Design and Layout	Jennie R. Bush of Designworks, Inc.
Photography and Illustration Direction	John Lemberg
Photography	Tim Boole, Steve Seeger, and Neill Whitlock of Photographers, Inc.
Styling	Jan Keeton
Makeup/Hair Styling	Gigi Coker Cindy Gregg
Illustration	Phil French

The Mary Kay Guide to Beauty was set in ITC Garamond and Vivaldi by DEKR Corporation of Woburn, Massachusetts. International Colour Services, Inc., of Rochester, New York, supplied the separations and camera work. The book was printed on 70-pound Warren Flokote Web paper from Lindenmeyr Paper Company of Boston, Massachusetts, at W. A. Krueger Company of New Berlin, Wisconsin.

Additional photo credits appear on page 240.

It is with great love, pride, and respect that we dedicate this book to all the beauty experts at Mary Kay Cosmetics—the over 200,000 independent beauty consultants who make up our organization. These remarkable women do so much more than teach skin care and makeup artistry. Each day they bring beauty into the lives of others, cheerfully giving of their time, knowledge, and experience.

Our beauty consultants are the reason Mary Kay Cosmetics has achieved so much in its first twenty years. Through their future efforts, millions of women (and maybe even a few men) will learn more about "beauty" in all its wonderful dimensions!

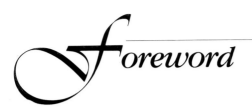oreword

Of all the lessons I've learned in the cosmetics business, one of the most universal is that women like to be told that they're beautiful. And why not? There's no nicer compliment. It's only natural that we feel better about ourselves when others offer their praise, support, and approval.

But did you ever stop to consider that the better you like yourself, the more beautiful you appear? It's a perpetual cycle: once you begin feeling your best — and believing that you are — you'll project that image to the world!

At Mary Kay Cosmetics, our goal has always been to help women bring the beauty they have inside them — outside! Instead of concentrating on what's less than perfect, we encourage them to look at the big picture — the positive qualities that make them special and unique. I don't know how many times I've heard a woman worry about her close-set eyes when she should have been focusing on their gorgeous shade of blue! It's not just coincidence that when you look past your shortcomings, others do too.

Still, that doesn't mean you can "wish" your way to an attractive appearance. Looking good takes motivation and effort. It means setting aside time to do those things that will contribute to your physical and your emotional well-being. Rule Number One: Include yourself on your list of priorities — no matter how long that list may be.

Believe me, I know how busy a typical day can be. There's your career, your family, your home, and dozens of other obligations. But stop and think how much better things seem to go on days when your energy level is high and you're feeling good about yourself. Somehow knowing you're in optimum form generates an unmistakable confidence, an attitude *and* assurance that can carry you through anything.

As for finding the time to devote to a sensible beauty routine, one of my favorite expressions is: You can do it! Just as work expands to fill the time available for it, you'll also be able to fit self-care and self-awareness into your daily life if you really want to. The key is not to think of this time as just an indulgence. Instead, consider it an important part of your life, necessary to keep you functioning in peak condition.

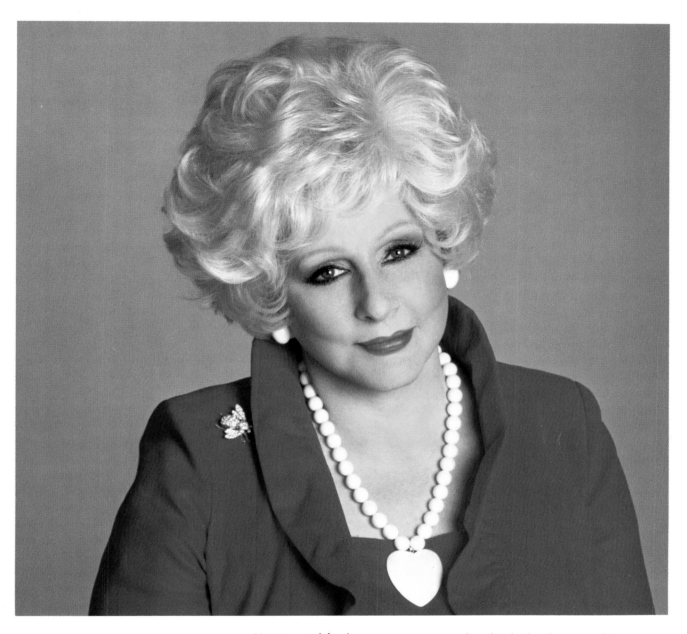

Yet inevitably there are women who think they're too old or too ugly or too unsuccessful ever to be beautiful. How wrong they are! Many's the time I've convinced a woman who felt that way just to try skin-care and beauty products. So often the results are magical. All of a sudden, that woman feels pretty — and it shows inside and out. From that point on, she becomes dedicated to her daily beauty routine.

This, of course, doesn't mean hours of fussing and primping. Nobody has that much time. Instead, I recommend a positive attitude and sense of self, discovering, step by step, exactly what makes *you* so special — and so beautiful.

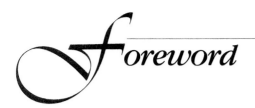
Foreword

There's that word again — *beautiful.* Don't let it scare you. There's no need, since today's definition is so different from what it used to be. Beauty now is both accessible and attainable, including such qualities as energy, health, and vitality, radiance, confidence, and personal style.

So how do you reach your beauty potential? First, you need an intelligent plan of action with challenging, but always realistic, goals. We at Mary Kay Cosmetics believe everyone can climb the ladder of success, provided she moves up one rung at a time. And once you understand that this pertains to all aspects of your life — from skin care to diet to career — you'll be able to reach new heights.

I also encourage you to experiment, to grow, learn, and keep pace with what's going on in fashion, makeup, your field, and your world. When you step outside your comfort zone, I know you'll find the results to be well worth the effort.

Still another necessary element of being your best is believing in yourself — capitalizing on your assets and making the most of your talents. Then decide what changes you want to make and what areas you'd most like to improve. Once you know what it takes to make you feel terrific — and believe it's possible — you can start a positive move in that direction.

Finally, be sure you take advantage of what the experts have to offer. Whatever you need — information, encouragement, motivation, advice — don't hesitate to turn to those who have the knowledge and experience to guide you.

This book was designed to be a working tool — a source for direction, facts, and inspiration. As you read it, bear in mind that beauty is individual and personal, that the look and feeling you're after is one with which you can be happy and comfortable each and every day of your life.

The first step is the hardest: making a commitment to yourself, *for* yourself. But once you do it, you're well on your way!

Mary Kay

$\mathcal{C}$ontents

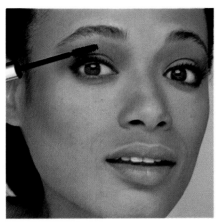

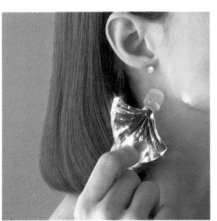

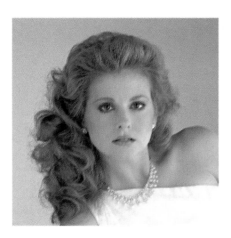

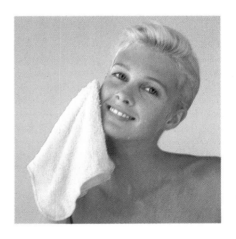

Your Special Beauty

Reflect on the real beauty within you that radiates to everyone you see. Your personal appeal begins with your view of yourself, the pleasure and joy you take in being who you are. Take a fresh, new look at yourself right now. Get to know and appreciate that special person. Then learn how to tap your inner beauty to create a personal style. Your beauty potential lies within.

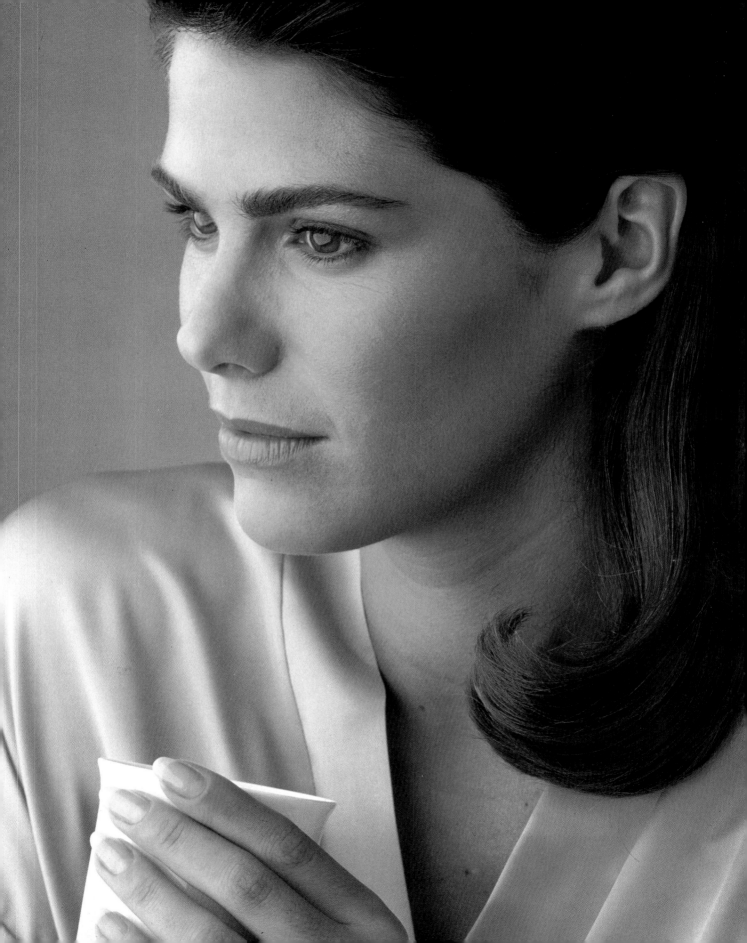

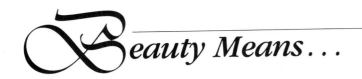

Beauty Means...

You can always tell when a woman feels beautiful. She has an extra bounce in her stride, a gleam in her eyes, and a sparkle in her smile. Even if you can't pinpoint the exact cause, a woman who feels beautiful has an aura that comes from within: a special confidence and charisma people can't help but notice. That's why a single set of beauty standards doesn't work anymore. Today, women are free to develop their own style, to set their own goals and priorities, to make the choices and changes that affect their lives. Most important of all, they have the freedom to fulfill their potential — to take control of both their looks and their lives.

Personal beauty evolves from the interest you take in yourself. It comes from having commitment, energy, and a sincere desire to be your best. Whether you're a student, a homemaker, a career woman, or a grandmother, you have to start by making space in your life for beauty: reserving time for yourself — not as a bonus or a special indulgence, but as a regular, important part of your daily routine. Whatever your lifestyle, you can set up an ongoing self-care regimen that suits your individual needs. The key is education — taking an intelligent, positive, and realistic approach to beauty. It means understanding how your body functions; why skin and hair care are so essential; and how to use cosmetics for maximum benefit.

The Mary Kay Guide to Beauty addresses these issues — and many others. It provides you with the information you want to complement your own motivation and the knowledge you need to bring about effective, long-lasting results. In addition, we ask you some eye-opening questions designed to help you take a closer look and see yourself in a new, and perhaps different, light. These inventories should spark your imagination and expand your outlook. They should help you evaluate what you like best about yourself and help you envision and realize your most important beauty goals.

Beauty is not so much hard work as it is a commitment and a willingness to invest in yourself. We think you'll find that a regular beauty routine is one of the surest investments you'll ever make — because you're responsible for the returns. In the following pages, we introduce you to an approach to beauty that is easy, enjoyable, and flexible enough for even the busiest schedules. The best part is the dividends are tremendous. You'll feel happier, more alive, and more attractive. And as a result, you *will* be!

Knowing who you are and how special you can be means taking an interest in yourself — learning everything you can about your personal style of beauty, from the inside out. It's a fresh new outlook that starts here and lasts a lifetime, a philosophy of self-care that helps you make the most of your own good looks.

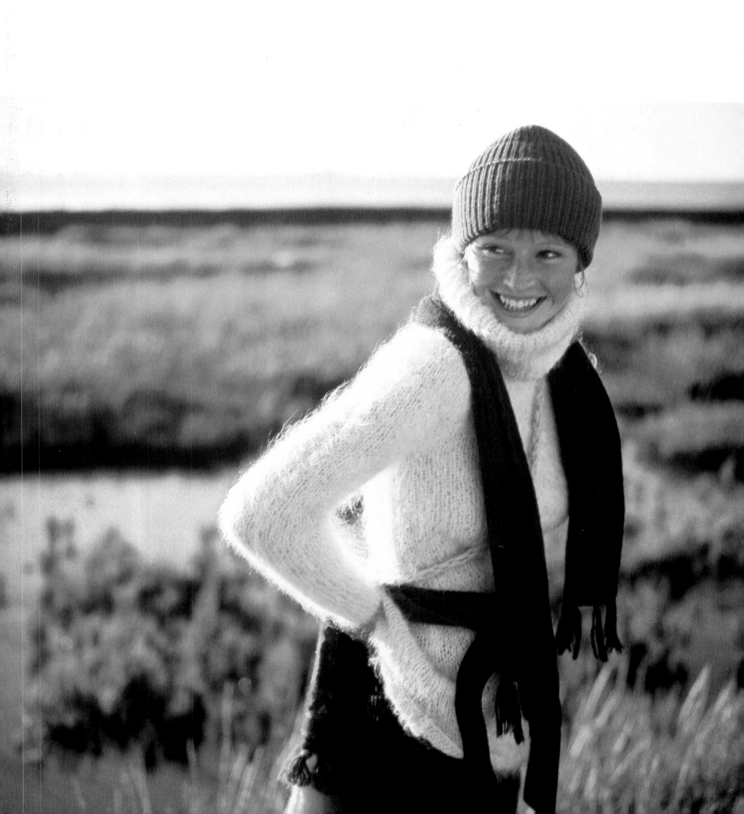

Important Basics

Every effective beauty plan should revolve around four important basics: skin care, glamour makeup, hair care, and a healthy, fit body. Together these elements contribute to your total look — which means each needs your special attention.

As you begin a routine, it may help to remember that beauty is an ongoing commitment for every woman. It calls for an active approach, based on positive, realistic actions and changes. You want it to be fun and exciting — something you look forward to. It shouldn't be complicated, time-consuming, or monotonous. The key is to look at the rewards: the luxury of devoting time to yourself, the confidence that goes hand in hand with looking your best, and the sheer pleasure of seeing the tangible benefits of your efforts.

There's no better feeling than knowing you're in peak condition. The more you learn, the more you want to learn. The more you accomplish, the higher you set your goals. You begin to welcome the responsibility of taking care of yourself — and, as a result, all your other responsibilities seem simpler and can be accomplished more smoothly.

Healthy, glowing *skin* is an essential part of any beauty look. Because your skin is unique, it takes more than mysterious lotions and creams to keep it looking radiant. It takes knowledge and a skin-care program based on products that work together to meet your special needs. In addition, you want to take full advantage of all the latest advances in scientific research and technology. In *The Mary Kay Guide to Beauty* we present five steps to beautiful skin: cleanse, stimulate, freshen, moisturize, and protect. By following this regimen and using the right products for your skin type, you can keep your complexion looking clear, fresh, and vibrant.

Next in your beauty routine is *glamour*. There's a wonderful feeling that naturally goes along with finding just the right makeup look and cosmetics. It could be a smoky, rich eye shadow, a sensational lip color, or a blush that gives you a sun-kissed glow. Glamour makeup can accentuate your best features. It also lets you enhance, define, color, and update your own special look. And with proper guidance, you can learn to camouflage and correct. Included in our glamour makeup section are tips and ideas for selecting cosmetics, as well as step-by-step instructions for creating the looks you desire to attain. In addition, you'll see how cosmetics can change the way

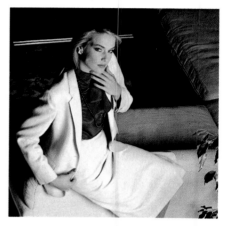

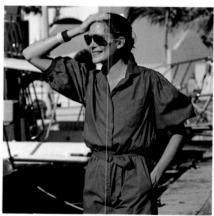

At work and at play, your beauty routine can make all the difference — clean, radiant skin; makeup that suits the occasion, your mood, and your unique style; shining, healthy hair; and a fit, toned body. The end result: a more beautiful you, every day.

When you put all the beauty basics together, the effect is naturally glowing — and yours alone. You've created your personal style by doing the most for yourself.

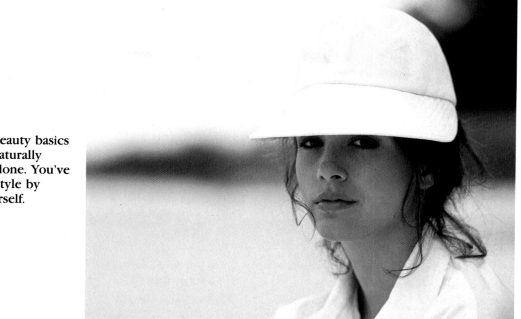

you feel about yourself — giving an important lift to both your appearance and your confidence.

Nothing enhances your glamorous image quite the way a flattering *hair* style can. For hair that is at its healthy best — clean, shiny, and manageable — you need a total, systematic approach to hair care. As with skin care, scientific developments have provided information to help you meet the individual needs of your hair type, whether it's dry, normal, or oily. Our hair-care section includes information on determining your hair type, along with guidelines for selecting the routine and hair-care products best suited to you. You'll find suggestions on style, cut, and color — which, with the advice of your hair stylist, will help you choose a look compatible with your hair type, face shape, personality, and lifestyle.

Finally, so many qualities of today's beauty look rely on a *body* that's toned, fit, and healthy. In addition to a basic program that shows you how to care for the skin all over your body, we show you how to get in shape with up-to-date information on exercise, relaxation, and all-around fitness. We also provide you with timeless, versatile wardrobe guidelines that will help you put together a look that is uniquely — and stylishly — yours.

The Mary Kay Guide to Beauty challenges you to develop your own personal beauty by instructing and inspiring you to become your very best. Use it as a guide to discover something new and beautiful about the way you look — and the way you *can* look.

Taking a Closer Look

Nothing does more for your appearance than feeling terrific. When you feel terrific, you possess a radiant glow and a healthy vitality. It's the way you look when something wonderful happens — when you're able to help someone, when you achieve a special goal, or when you're around those you love. Your inner beauty can't help but shine through.

Being beautiful becomes a total experience, a combination of the physical, the emotional, and the psychological. Many factors come into play — from the sparkle in your eyes to your easy, natural smile; from your genuine laugh to your graceful walk and confident posture. These features distinguish total beauty from just a pretty face. They help every woman look and feel her beautiful best.

The most effective beauty plans start from the inside. Like most clichés, "Beauty is more than skin deep" is true. It can be most beneficial to take time to think about your inner strengths — the many qualities that make you beautiful from within. You'll be better equipped to evaluate what you like most about yourself and what you might like to improve. The following inventory can help you start making these decisions. It was designed to put things in perspective, to help you honestly assess areas for change and growth, and to guide you in setting realistic goals and objectives.

Today, being beautiful calls for action, not perfection. The key is knowing what's important to you — what you want out of life — and accepting the challenge to become the best person you can be.

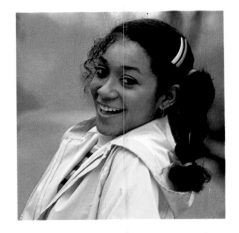

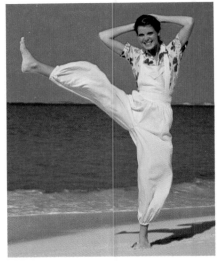

Vitality comes from within and gives your look that extra sparkle. Who you are shows beautifully in the way you look and the way others see you.

Read the statements below when you have time to relax and give them your complete attention. Look at yourself objectively and try not to think about how others might evaluate you. Circle those statements you feel best describe your strong points. Circle as many, or as few, as you like. Then turn to pages 18 and 19. Remember, this isn't a test, and no one can fail!

1. I'm good at helping people around me feel comfortable.
2. I have respect for who I am and what I do.
3. I don't compare myself to others, and I enjoy being me.
4. I feel sure of myself when I'm with others.
5. I feel that I'm a loving person who enjoys getting close to people.
6. I'm loyal to my friends, and I can be there for them if they need me.
7. My feelings toward my family members are warm, supportive, and understanding.
8. I enjoy the opposite sex and am comfortable in their company.
9. I like to give 100 percent of myself to projects I consider important.
10. I can rely on my personal or religious beliefs for courage when I need it.

11. When the going gets tough, I can keep going.
12. I'm able to recover from disappointments.
13. I set realistic goals and fulfill them.
14. I can determine what's most important to me and give those things my best attention.
15. I don't have to rely on others to start up new projects.
16. I'm open to other opinions, but I have confidence in my own ideas.
17. I'm capable of getting things done in cooperation with others.
18. I have my own interests outside my family and/or work.
19. I'm curious about the world around me, and I try to stay well informed.
20. I take an interest in some form of artistic expression that reflects my own, or another, culture.
21. I try to appreciate people who are quite different from me and learn from them.
22. I strive for my own personal success.
23. I use my time well, balancing my work responsibilities with personal interests.
24. I find the time and energy for the things I really want to do, both for myself and for others.
25. I laugh easily, and I like to make others laugh.
26. Even in bad times, I can laugh at myself.

27. I would describe myself as a giving and sympathetic person.
28. I enjoy sharing.
29. I feel confident that I can shape my own world and create a good future for myself.
30. I adjust to situations that aren't exactly what I'm used to.
31. I handle surprises, good or bad, well.
32. It's easy for me to feel excited about interesting new places, people, and projects.
33. When I feel something is wrong, I do my best to try to correct it.
34. Whatever my religious convictions, I have faith in the potential for good in humanity and in the world.
35. I don't expect my life to be perfect, but I tend to concentrate on what's good in it.
36. I feel positive about where my life is going.
37. I like the way I look, and I'm interested in exploring new ways of being attractive.

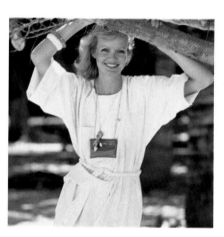

Discovering Yourself

Everyone has individual strengths and weaknesses. But by getting to know yourself better you can determine where you want to make changes. You can also establish ambitions, goals, and routines that coincide with your capabilities and lifestyle.

Because the way you see yourself and the way you look are inseparable, your special traits are reflected in your appearance and your image. The inventory statements have been grouped below to relate to several specific character traits that affect the outward expression of your inner personality. See which ones reflect your current strengths — and which ones are traits you'd like to work on.

Statements 1, 2, 3, and 4 relate to your *self-confidence* — your poise and ease with others, as well as your pride in yourself. If you circled any of these statements, your self-confidence is probably expressed in your facial expression and body movement. Self-confidence gives you a special radiance that shines in your eyes and imparts an added sense of self-esteem to your appearance.

If you identified with numbers 5 through 8, you have a high capacity for *intimacy*, and you are a good friend, an excellent family member, and popular in social gatherings. The inner quality of intimacy shows through in the way you look at people and speak to them. You maintain eye contact with people you're talking to, and you let your looks express your true nature so that people can get close to you.

If you found items 9 through 12 to be true, you rate high on *inner strength* and are more capable than most of seeing projects through. High energy and stamina are the virtues of people who have strength, and these qualities add an aura of power to the way you look.

Statements 13 through 17 relate to your sense of *direction*. If you circled these statements, it means you know how to set priorities and goals *and* fulfill them. You're independent and secure, and you like taking the initiative. Well-directed people radiate assurance and self-awareness; having a purposeful attitude toward your life can give your posture an extra lift and your entire physical appearance a genuine, straightforward beauty.

Numbers 18 through 21 relate to your *versatility*, showing that you're a person who is interested in the world around you, that you are outgoing and knowledgeable. Your versatility adds sparkle to

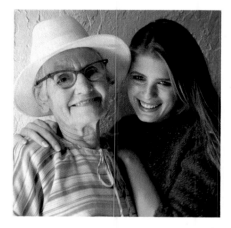

The real beauty of friendship is that it's ageless and timeless. Nothing makes you shine the way genuine loving and caring for others can.

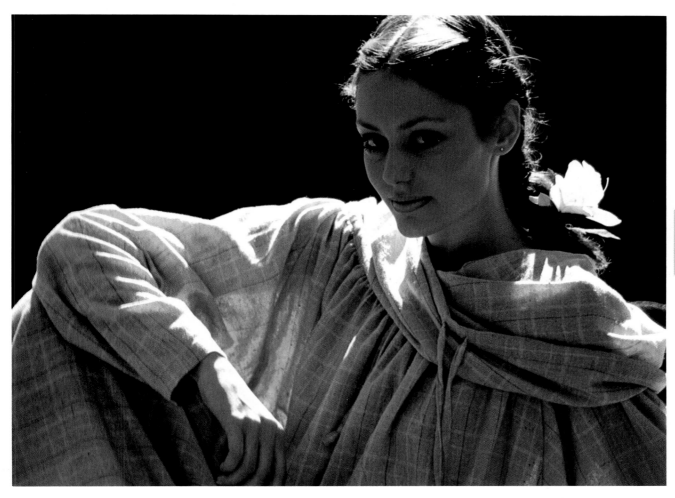

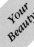

Your many expressions and moods — pensive, happy, loving — show you're comfortable being yourself. A positive, healthy self-image is an essential beauty asset, a number-one priority for looking your radiant best.

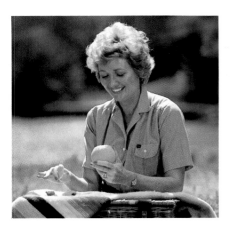

your looks because your sincere interest in people, places, and things endows your beauty with the lively glow of an active mind.

Sentences 22 through 24 are about your *self-fulfillment*, your interest in success, and your ability to achieve. Your capacity to fulfill yourself as much as possible adds the quality of serene confidence to the way you look and gives your appearance its special note of self-assurance.

The last thirteen statements, numbers 25 through 37, relate to your *attitude* — how you feel about yourself, your life, and the world around you. If you thought these ideas expressed your view of life, you are positive, optimistic, and enthusiastic — all high-energy qualities that give your looks extra impact. Your attitude is also reflected in your generosity, flexibility, and ability to adapt when necessary, as it is in your charity and sense of humor. These characteristics show up in the way you treat yourself and others.

Inner beauty is where total beauty begins. If you feel good about yourself, you'll look better, too. Read on. You'll find lots of ideas for making your inner beauty work for you — today and for the rest of your life.

Self-Confidence

Self-confidence is a quality that's *essential* to how attractive you are and how attractive you feel.

Self-confidence comes from knowing, and liking, who you are. It allows you to be yourself, to hold your own in everything you do.

Having confidence in yourself shows in your poised self-assurance — the way you have of making everyone around you feel good (because *you* feel so good!). It comes from taking pride in yourself and what you do. Self-confidence is simply self-esteem — appreciating yourself and *showing it!*

One of the best ways to boost your self-confidence is to learn how to enjoy yourself. That means more than having a good time with others. It means concentrating on what's best about you, and taking on the challenge of accomplishing what you want to change about yourself.

Self-confidence also means self-respect — respect for your body, your mind, and your spirit. That comes from taking good care of yourself. Staying healthy so your body functions well. Staying alert to the world around you to keep your mind in shape. Staying true to yourself to keep your spirit wholesome. Respecting who you are sometimes means standing up for your beliefs and ideas — and learning how to do it gracefully.

Self-confidence comes from your ability to concentrate on yourself — not in a selfish, narcissistic way, but in a way that allows you to be aware of both your gifts and your shortcomings. If you think positively about your own strengths, you aren't tempted to measure yourself against someone else. There will always be someone who can outdo you at something. Having self-confidence means recognizing that no one else is quite like you, and that it is therefore pointless to compare yourself to others. It doesn't mean being blind to your faults. It means being in touch with your best inner self. It means trusting yourself, and believing that you can be the kind of person you want to be.

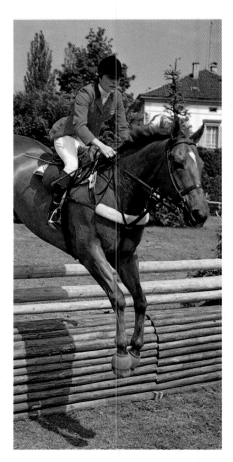

You take on new challenges and expect the best because you *know* you can do it. Your faith in yourself gives you energy, strength, verve — the confidence you need to create your individual style of beauty.

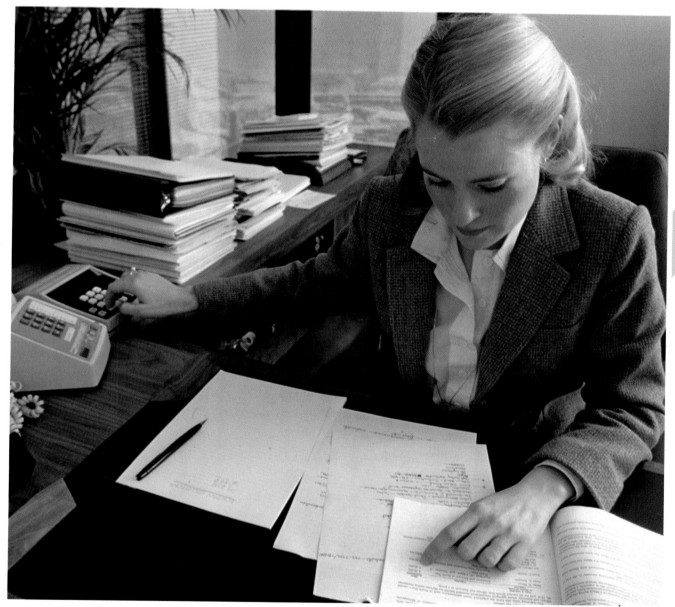

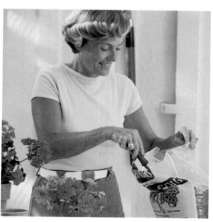

Self-confidence is your key to personal success. You believe in yourself and trust your abilities. You understand and appreciate your unique qualities. There's no one else quite like you.

Intimacy

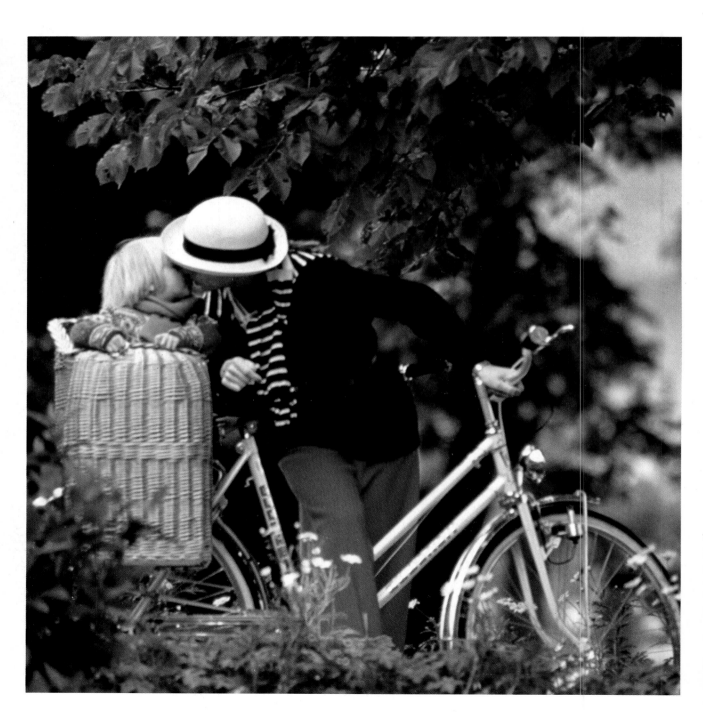

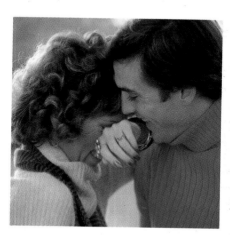

The ability to get close, to understand and listen, to love — that's what intimacy is. Your personal warmth gives you a glow that embraces everyone around you and makes them feel as good as you do.

Intimacy is that special capacity you have for getting close to people, for getting involved in what's important.

Intimacy is personal warmth; it comes from your ability to open up and let others know exactly who you are. Intimacy is sharing yourself — giving your all to your family and friends, getting close to the people who are meaningful in your life. And, of course, it can mean falling in love.

Intimacy means having the courage to get involved . . . with the special people you love, and with the rest of your world. Your ability to be intimate comes from your attitude toward people in general. When you understand your own needs, you are open to responding to human needs all around you. You can give everything you do that little bit extra because you want to, and because getting close to people is important to you.

You can develop your capacity for intimacy simply by being a warm and caring friend, by being an understanding parent and family member, by looking for ways to make all your relationships closer and more meaningful. Sometimes it means a gesture — a phone call to a sick friend or a present for a special birthday. Often, though, it simply means being a good listener and having a good heart. You'll find opportunities to develop intimacy every day if you look for them.

People who are capable of intimacy are people we love. We trust them with our feelings because they have trusted us with theirs. We can tell them our problems and know they'll try to understand. We can laugh easily with them because we know they take sincere pleasure in our joy. We can even cry with them because we know they are not afraid of their own emotions, or of ours.

Intimacy means not being afraid of who you are, and wanting to share yourself with the people you love. It means being able to love — and be loved.

Inner Strength

Inner strength is your faith in yourself and your own abilities, the power you have within you to make good things happen and to bounce back when disappointments come.

Inner strength is a kind of internal energy; it can come from your relationships, from your religion, or from your commitment to make the most of who you are. It gives you the potential to strive for excellence and achieve it, to hold on to your convictions and apply them to everything you do, to be strong for others as well as for yourself.

Sometimes, it's easier to *appear* to be strong than it is to really *be* strong within. No matter what the circumstances, inner strength is derived from what you possess internally: your faith in yourself, the responsibility you feel toward the people who love you, your standards and beliefs — your character.

Inner strength comes from having learned how to deal with mistakes, misunderstandings, and even bad luck. It means learning how to work out whatever may go wrong — from a stalled car to a major family crisis.

When you're strong internally, you can count on yourself and others can count on you, too. You take responsibility for yourself and know how to shoulder your own burdens. And, when the people who are important to you need your help, they know they can rely on you.

Having inner strength means being a self-starter, a person who can initiate difficult new projects without the help of others. Inner strength also gives you the emotional wisdom and the internal energy to start again when those projects sometimes fail.

Inner strength is the power you have inside you to cope with the worst as well as the best; to take on the world with optimism whatever it brings; to take risks without fear of failure; and to accept failure by learning from it.

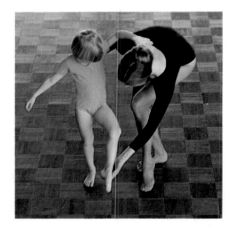

Your capacity to share — to pass on to family and friends what you know and love —- gives special meaning to your life. Others know they can rely on you because you know you can rely on yourself.

Inner strength gives your life direction. It means being a self-starter and having the initiative, energy, and determination to accomplish your goals and fulfill your needs.

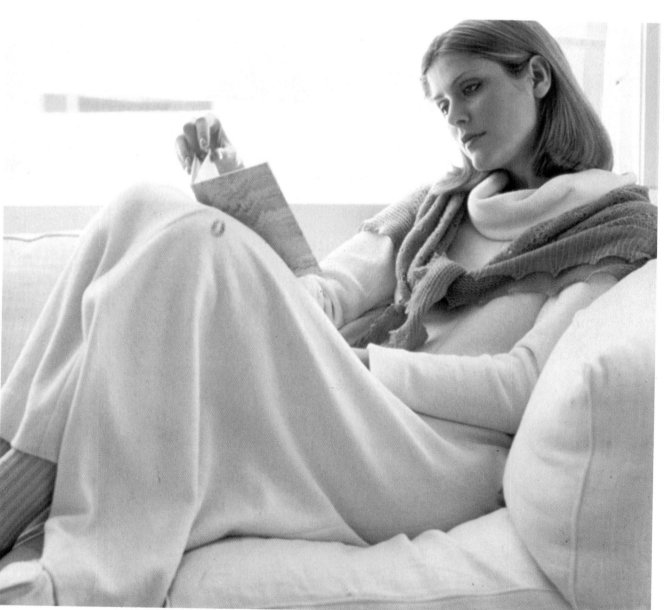

Versatility

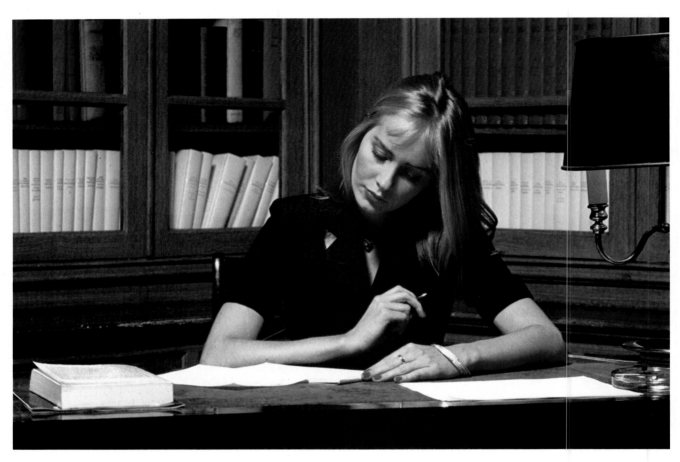

Because of your versatility, you not only are open to new ideas — you enjoy the unfamiliar and the unexpected. You take the time to cultivate your interests and are able to meet new challenges with confidence.

Versatility means taking an interest in your world and exploring its many facets, finding what fascinates you and developing your own special talents.

Versatility is an expansive outlook on everything around you, the ability to go beyond your life's boundaries to discover new interests. It comes from cultivating an appreciation of people, places, and ideas that are different or unfamiliar to you, and it gives you the desire to learn as much as you can from every situation, and to expand your life beyond its everyday horizons.

Versatility means acquiring an adventurous perspective on being alive; reaching out to embrace the new; excelling in a variety of personal skills; being curious and informed; viewing the universe as a bountiful source of wonder in which you want to be involved.

Being versatile means developing more than one dimension of yourself — not locking yourself into any one role or mold, and not limiting yourself to rigid restrictions imposed on you by others or by yourself.

You can develop versatility by expanding your own expectations of yourself, by going beyond what you know you can do well to discover new and challenging areas of yourself. You become versatile when you take the time to cultivate your own potential interests. Whether it involves learning to knit an afghan or accepting a job promotion, versatility helps you meet challenges with confidence.

Being versatile will also make you feel better about yourself. Absorbing new information and being curious about the world will make you more interesting, more animated. You'll find you have more to say to people — at home, at parties, or on the job. Reading the newspaper every day, attending classes at the Y, or simply teaching yourself a new skill are all part of versatility.

When you're versatile, you are open to all that's new and exciting. You appreciate people who are different from you because you know you can learn from them. You're capable of adapting to the unfamiliar and you're comfortable with yourself in almost any situation.

Versatility offers you an introduction to as many situations, places, and people as you find interesting; it gives you the ability to play as hard as you work, and to discover the very best in yourself and your world.

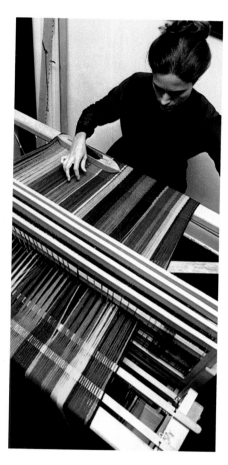

You take advantage of every opportunity to learn, and you find new experiences appealing. You appreciate insights others share; they help you see your world in a new and different light.

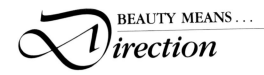

Direction

Having direction is setting your own goals and striving for them, knowing what your priorities are and giving them primary attention. It's taking the initiative getting projects started, moving toward what you want, and feeling secure about where you want to go.

Having direction is approaching your life with the sound conviction that your aims are realistic and achievable. It comes from your ability to concentrate on what's important and to dedicate your energy to your most meaningful goals. It's having a sense of purpose.

Having direction means taking the straightforward path toward your destinations, being sure of where you're headed because you know your goals are right for you. And sometimes it means taking a less traveled, more difficult road because it's the only one that can take you to exactly where you want to be. A strong sense of direction can help you be a better friend and parent. Sometimes we use direction for personal goals — to start a new career or lose weight, for example. It takes a lot of energy to do either, and a good sense of inner direction can help you channel that energy to achieve the best results. Living your life with a sense of direction involves having a strong sense of who you are and what you want.

You can put direction into your life by defining your most important goals: the areas in which you want to excel, the milestones you're confident you can attain. Do you want to go back to school? Be a more patient listener? Climb the corporate ladder? Direction is what keeps you moving forward.

Direction gives you the ability to shape your own future. It gives purpose and an overall design to your everyday activities. Direction gives you a perspective on almost everything you do, and helps you understand how to get where you want to go.

When you have a clear sense of direction, you are willing to consider the many different roads that can lead to your destination. You are willing to be patient while determining the very best course for realizing your ambitions.

Believing in your dreams and planning ways to make them come true gives you direction. So does taking yourself and your goals seriously. Having direction means paying attention to what really matters to you and disregarding unimportant distractions. It means having confidence in yourself and your abilities.

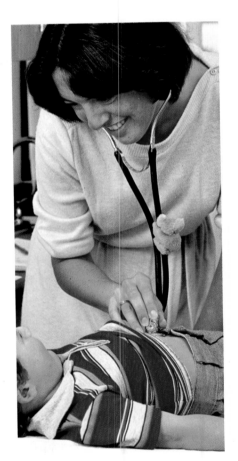

You strive for what you want because your goals are important to you and you know you can achieve them. Your sense of direction adds structure and meaning to your life; it gives you purpose and strength, the determination you need to get what you want.

The beauty of giving your all to make your dreams come true is that fantasies *can* become reality; you'll find that your highest aims are within your grasp when you're willing to reach for them.

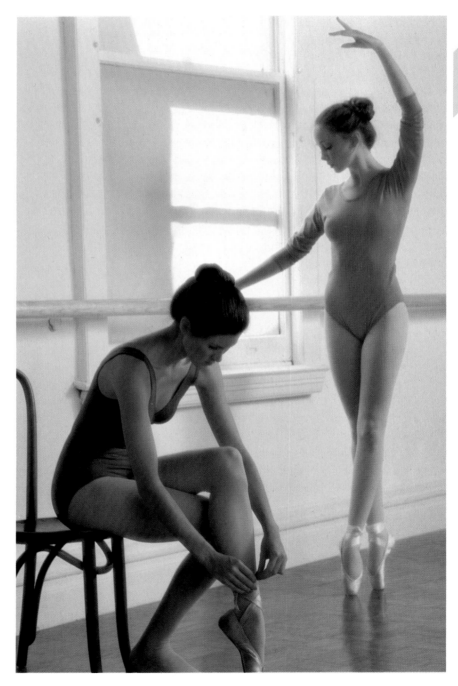

Self-Fulfillment

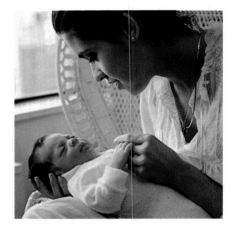

Self-fulfillment is your commitment to achievement in every area of your life. It's an ability to devote everything you have to doing your best and your sense of balance in deciding what success means to you — both personally and in your work life.

Self-fulfillment is what your goals are based on, the reason you strive to achieve them. It's understanding yourself, your needs and desires, and how you can best accomplish them. It's orienting your world toward attaining your own personal satisfaction, as well as being aware of the fulfillment you can derive from others.

Self-fulfillment means having a healthy awareness that only you can really make yourself happy. Fulfilling yourself begins with understanding what makes you feel best about yourself and your life. It comes from knowing who you are in relation to the world around you. It helps you make the right decisions, based on your own self-knowledge.

Self-fulfillment means developing a clear sense of what's really rewarding to you — not only the outward appearances of success, but emotional gratification as well. It also means putting all the elements of your life — work, family, and friends — into a balanced perspective. You have to know what makes you feel best. You could be as fulfilled by a simple, private activity that's meaningful to you as by receiving public acclaim. Fulfillment is very personal, and specifically related to what you alone want from life. Sometimes it involves compromise, trading off a career for children, or a promotion for a job you like better.

Being self-fulfilled gives you a spirit of generosity: when you know what makes you feel good, you want to share it with others, and you want to help them fulfill themselves.

Self-fulfillment requires energy and commitment. What really fulfills you may not be easily attainable, or the challenge itself may offer you the most fulfillment. Fulfilling yourself isn't always easy, but it's always worth the effort.

You treasure those moments that give you so much happiness — simple pleasures that reward and enrich your life. Self-fulfillment comes from the smallest task done well or from a challenging project finally completed. It's a feeling of satisfaction that comes from achieving what you set out to do.

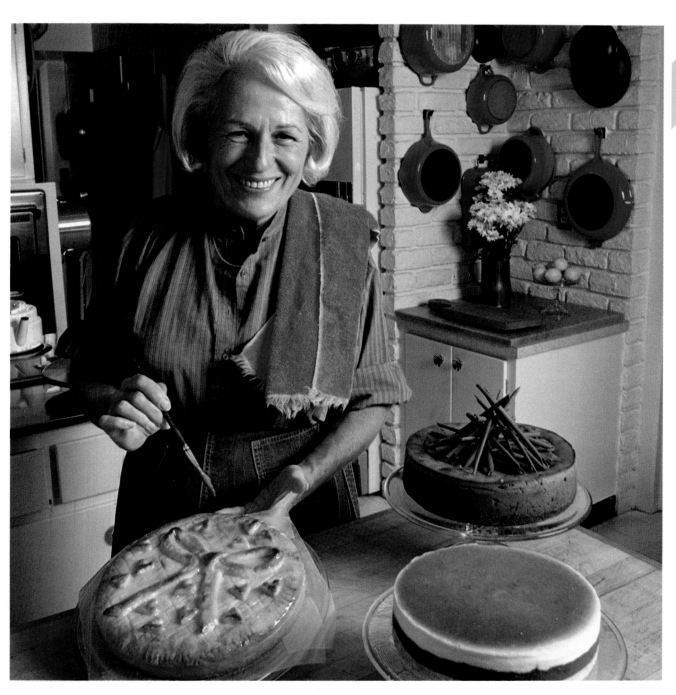

Positive Attitude

A positive attitude is represented by your positive perspective on yourself and all of life around you, your enthusiasm for what excites you, and your optimism for the kind of future you know you can create. It's your compassion and generosity, your ability to change when change is for the good, and a sense of humor that becomes your saving grace in the worst of times.

Attitude is the source of your whole personality — the way you see the world and the way the world sees you. When you have a healthy, positive attitude you know how to apply constructive intelligence to your problems as well as your goals; your self-assurance allows you to enjoy being you; your fine-tuned self-awareness both perceives and expresses what you know to be right and good.

A positive attitude means having an outgoing involvement in yourself and the people you care about, a day-by-day joy in making the most of whatever life brings you — not complaining about what life fails to bring you. A positive attitude comes from your personal enthusiasm, your wholehearted zest for the life and people you love.

Being positive means looking for the potential in even the worst situations. It's approaching each day knowing that everything can't always be perfect, but believing that there is good to be found almost everywhere, and knowing you have the ability to try to change what you feel is wrong.

Optimism is the source of a positive attitude, and optimism comes from your own intelligent perspective on your capacity to make things better. When you believe in your own self-worth, you also believe in discovering what is worthwhile in everyone around you, and you look for the best in others.

A positive attitude gives you sincere enthusiasm for what really excites you, and allows you to become exuberantly involved in all your interests. It makes you the kind of person who can give others the strength and confidence to persevere in the worst of times, and even to laugh when everything goes wrong.

Having a positive attitude means finding joy and delight wherever they exist, and discovering them in unlikely places. The sources of a positive attitude are faith in humanity's potential for good and a sound belief in your own possibilities for excellence.

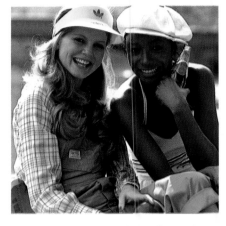

Your positive attitude makes others glad to be around you; your optimism is contagious. You feel good about your world because you feel so good about yourself — and that makes others feel good, too. There's always a bright side, and you know how to find it.

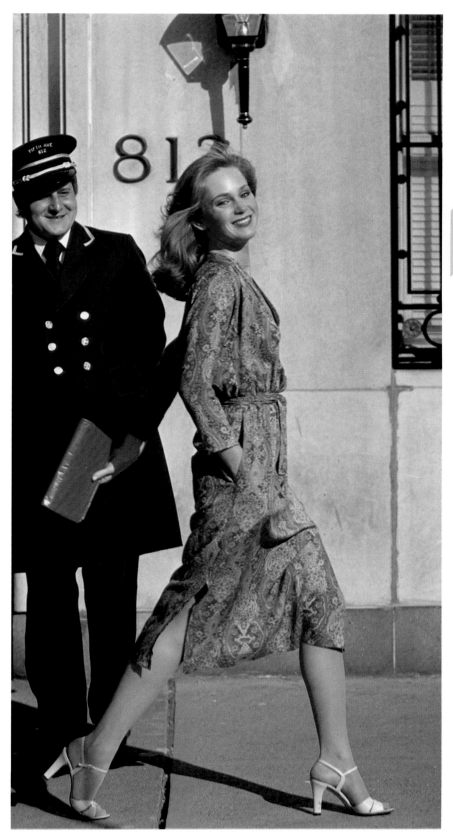

Your enthusiasm, energy, and confidence show through in everything you do. Others can't help noticing that something special about you when you look and feel your best.

Looking Good

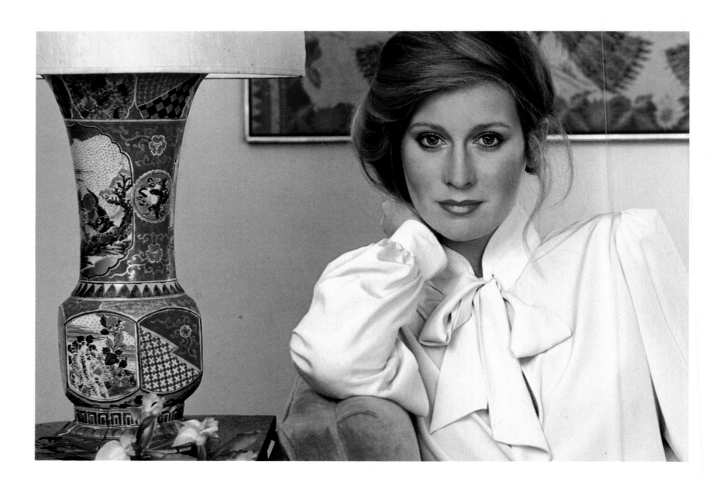

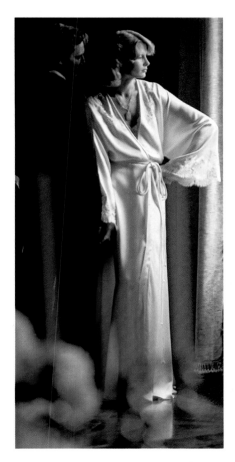

Your special beauty is yours alone. It comes from not only knowing but liking who you are. The time, thought, and energy you invest in understanding and enhancing yourself are worth the effort; the reward is that you bring the beauty you feel inside, outside.

Looking good — it means presenting the most attractive person you are capable of being to the world around you and taking an interest in your appearance. It's putting energy into what you look like and making yourself glow with all the qualities of inner beauty you know you possess.

Looking good is making the most of what is uniquely yours — not comparing yourself to others, but rejoicing in your own beauty. It's discovering the special allure that belongs to you alone — and making the *very most of it.*

Looking good means consistently doing what is best for you, establishing the best beauty habits and taking care of yourself because you know it matters: because you know *you* matter, and you want the world to know it too!

Looking good is letting your inner beauty radiate outward, presenting yourself to the world as a woman who knows what's beautiful about herself.

Looking good is paying attention to your appearance because you know it's important, and because it's so closely related to the way you feel about yourself. It's taking the time to express who you are in the way you look.

Good looks come from taking the time to understand the effect your appearance has on the people you deal with every day, from putting energy into adopting the right beauty habits. What fun it is to have someone cast an admiring eye on you, or smile when you walk into a room. Looking good is realizing your potential for being at your best in every sense.

Looking good starts with taking good care of yourself, learning as much as you can about making the most of how you appear to others. It's projecting the best of who you are onto the way you look every day. Whether getting ready to go to work or preparing for a special evening, you know how good it feels to look your best, and the way your inner feelings show up in your outward appearance makes all the difference.

Looking good is feeling good about who you are and glowing with your own special beauty.

Making It Yours

How do you take advantage of your special beauty? By putting your energy and caring into a presentation of yourself that radiates what's most beautiful from within. It shows on the outside in the polish and sparkle that come from taking the best possible care of your appearance.

Making it yours is using all your resources to make the most of yourself. It's creating a balance between who you are inwardly and how good you look outwardly. It's taking all the elements of your inner beauty and letting them shine through, adding a special sparkle to your eyes, projecting energy into your stride, giving a warm, healthy glow to your skin and a special graceful charm to your expression.

Making it yours means knowing what you have, understanding your potential, and taking an interest in developing it fully. Making it yours is what this book is about — taking the most advanced, effective, and efficient beauty techniques available and making them as much a part of you as your most beautiful inner qualities.

Your *self-confidence*: the special quality of knowing and liking yourself, an element of who you are that shows up beautifully in every expression and movement. Your capacity for *intimacy*: the personal warmth that adds a very special glow to the way you look. Your *inner strength*: the sense of wholesome energy that gives your looks dynamic power. Your *versatility*: the extra sparkle you get from having many facets to your personality. Your sense of *direction*: the positive motivation that animates your person. Your *self-fulfillment*: the way your contentment with yourself gives you an extra aura of beauty. Your *positive attitude*: the expression of your prettiest feature, your smile. *Looking good*: your ability to find what's best about who you are and let it show beautifully.

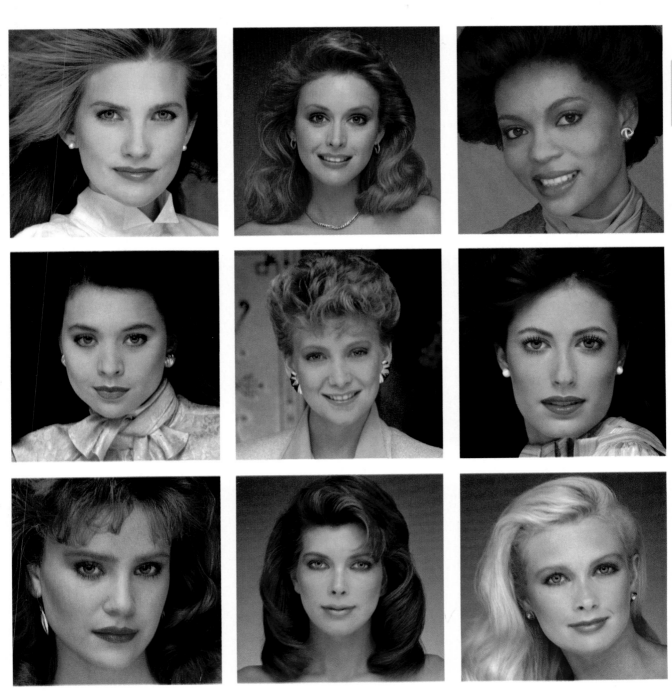

Skin Care

Total beauty begins with beautiful skin that is clean, fresh, and glowing. Your skin reflects the special care and knowledge you invest in your health, your state of mind, and your appearance. Well-cared-for skin is the basis of your overall beauty plan and your personal style. It's time to make successful skin care a goal — to learn how to achieve and maintain a soft, smooth, and radiant complexion.

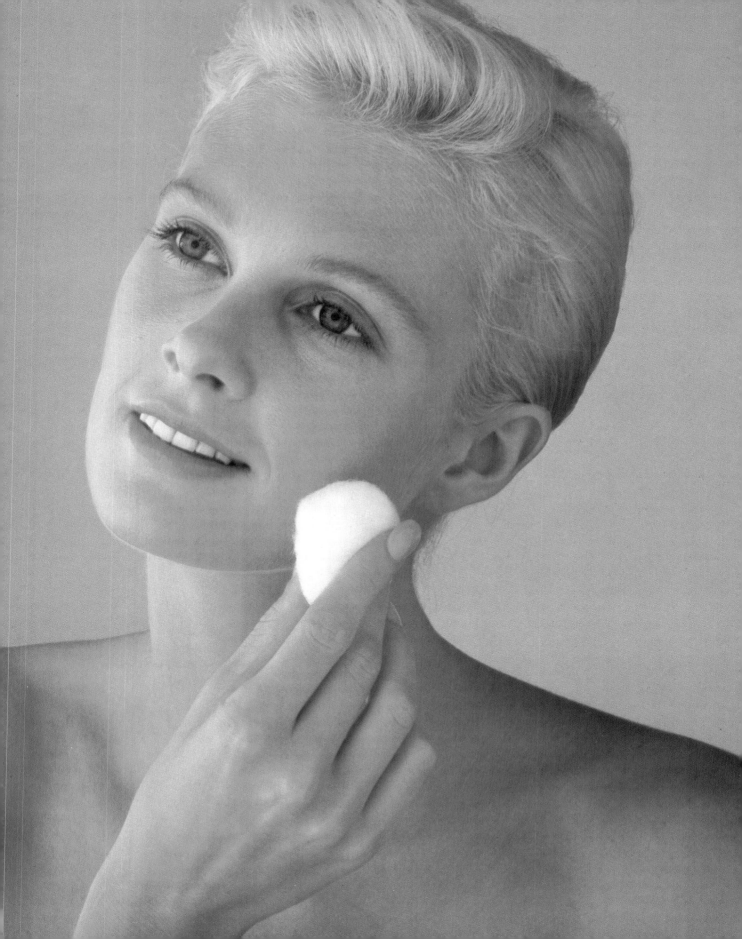

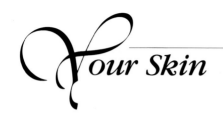

Your Skin

Beauty may begin within, but a personalized skin-care program can enhance your physical beauty. To make any skin-care program work for you, you must understand the nature of your skin: what it is; how it functions; why it looks and feels as it does.

Few people realize that skin is the largest organ of the body. Through it you experience the sense of touch and feel temperature, texture, and pressure. Your skin, a sensitive organ, is vital to your entire physiological system; it helps to keep your body temperature normal, which in turn keeps your internal organs functioning as they should. Your skin protects your body from harmful foreign substances, harmful bacteria, and some of the damaging ultraviolet rays from the sun. It also helps retain essential body fluids and heals most of its own wounds.

Your skin has a highly specialized two-layer structure that is constantly regenerating itself. The *epidermis* is its outermost layer — the layer of skin you see. It is composed of flat, dead skin cells that contain the protein keratin, plus a deeper layer of living cells. In healthy skins these living cells move to the surface of the skin in a continual four-week cycle. There they form a protective outer layer called the *stratum corneum.* As new cells are generated in the lower level of the epidermis, the top older cells harden, die, and are then shed from the surface steadily in microscopic flakes.

The upper layer of the epidermis acts as a barrier to prevent the entry of harmful bacteria into the lower, more vulnerable levels of skin, where infections can occur. This layer also slows the rate of moisture loss from lower layers of the skin. Harsh soaps or detergents can irritate skin by damaging the protective barrier and removing oils from the surface of the skin.

Beneath this paper-thin epidermis is a layer of skin, fifteen to forty times thicker than the epidermis, called the *dermis.* The dermis is composed of collagen and elastin fibers that support the vital components of the skin — the blood vessels, nerves, sweat glands, hair follicles, and sebaceous (oil) glands. *Fibrocytes,* cells that produce the collagen fibers, are also found in the dermis.

Many blood vessels and capillaries supply nutrients and oxygen to the skin. These *blood vessels* also help keep body temperature at a healthy level by contracting and expanding in response to external stimuli. When you are suddenly frightened, for example, your facial

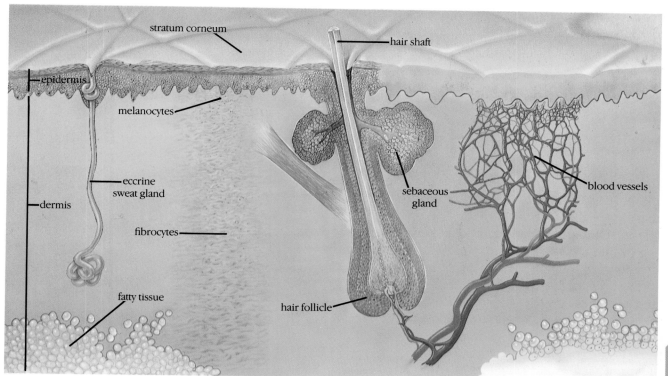

stratum corneum

hair shaft

epidermis

melanocytes

eccrine
sweat gland

sebaceous
gland

blood vessels

dermis

fibrocytes

fatty tissue

hair follicle

Below your skin's surface is an intricate system composed of many parts.

skin blanches. The blood vessels in your dermis contract, directing the blood (which helps supply color to your face) away from your skin and toward your body's tensed muscles. On the other hand, when you become overly warm from exertion, the blood vessels in your dermis expand so that heat from the center of your body moves to the outside, normalizing body temperature. In the process, skin tends to redden.

The most common sweat glands, the *eccrine glands,* also help control body temperature. These glands look like small coiled tubes that extend up through the epidermis and open onto the surface of the skin as pores. Sweat glands constantly bring small amounts of water (mixed with salt and waste products such as urea) to the surface of the skin. When the weather is very hot, or when your body becomes very warm, greater amounts of water are transported to the sweat pores, where the perspiration evaporates and cools the surface of your skin to prevent your body from overheating.

Hair grows in *hair follicles,* tubes located throughout the dermal layer of the skin. On animals, hair serves a protective function. On man, only eyelashes and eyebrows protect by shielding eyes from foreign substances. (Eyelashes, like the hair on your scalp, are shed and replaced regularly. Occasional loss of lashes should not be cause for alarm.)

The *sebaceous glands* — the source of the skin's natural oil supply — are attached to the hair follicles. They produce an oily substance called sebum, which they secrete to the follicles and onto

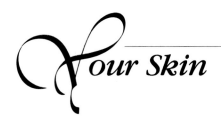

*Y*our *Skin*

the hair shafts for distribution over the skin's surface. Sebum coats the outermost layer of the skin, and is thought to help keep skin soft and pliable.

The sebum, in combination with surface moisture, forms a coating on the top layer of skin. Normally at an acidic pH level, this coating may help prevent bacterial infections. It may also contribute to the protective barrier function of the epidermis. The moisture and oil supply on the skin's surface is constantly replenished; therefore, cosmetic and skin-care products with a pH balance slightly different from that of the skin do not usually disturb its natural protective coating for a significant period of time.

At the lower levels of the epidermis, and to some extent at the very top of the dermal layer, *melanocytes* — cells containing the pigment melanin — give skin its color. The size of melanin granules produced by the cells and the amount of melanin within them determine the shade — light, medium, or dark — and/or consistency of the skin's pigmentation. Skin color is principally hereditary, but the melanocytes can be influenced by several factors over time, such as pregnancy or exposure to the sun. Freckles are concentrated melanin that accumulates in small patches.

Below the dermis, a layer of fatty tissue gives the skin its shape and insulates the body against extreme temperature changes, absorbs some physical trauma, and serves as a reservoir of energy. There is generally very little of this fatty tissue under facial skin; most of what's there is located in the chin and cheek areas.

Also underlying the dermis are muscles that connect it to the bones of the skull. We use muscles to form various facial expressions — smiling, frowning, and squinting. Some of the muscles perform involuntary movements, such as blinking. (Even when our faces are relatively still, the small muscles underlying the facial surface remain somewhat tense to hold the shape of the face.)

The facial surface does not retain the contours and lines of every expression because of elasticity — a property of the collagen and elastin fibers in the dermis. Elasticity is also affected by water in the epidermis. Dry skin, which may be insufficiently supplied with moisture and oil, however, may retain these small expression lines

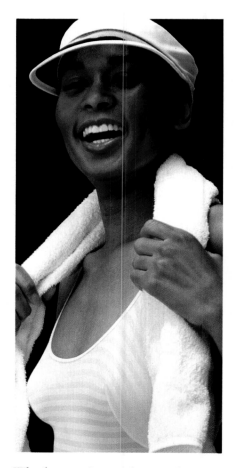

Whether you're awake or asleep, your skin performs its functions twenty-four hours a day. Proper skin care is vital to the health and appearance of your skin.

Healthy skin is essential to looking good. The more you know about what your skin is and what it does, the better you can make it look and feel.

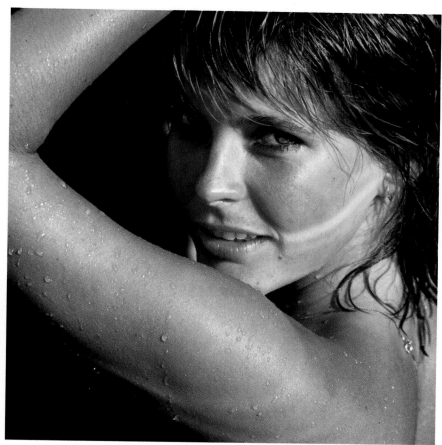

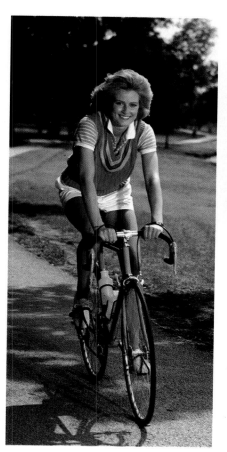

more easily than other skin types. Facial expressions are one of the principal causes (along with exposure to the sun) of the deeper wrinkling of the skin.

The goal of proper skin care, as outlined in the pages to come, is to keep your skin functioning at peak performance, to make it look and feel soft, smooth, and beautiful. A good skin-care routine can supplement the natural processes that keep your skin healthy and vibrant. The result: a naturally beautiful you!

Special Considerations

Skin is a highly responsive organ. It reacts to the internal changes in your body, as well as to the environment around you. The condition of your skin can change in response to some of these internal and external considerations, so it is sometimes necessary to modify your normal skin-care routine to accommodate such factors as age, hormonal influences, and environment.

Age The most significant change in your skin as you grow older occurs in the dermis. The sebaceous glands may become less active and produce less oil. Poorly lubricated skin may not retain water as easily, and as a result, your facial surface may dry out. You should remember to use foundations and moisturizers more frequently to prevent your skin from looking and feeling tight. If your skin has been oily throughout your lifetime, the visible effects of aging will be minimized. If your skin has always been dry, the dehydration that accompanies aging will be more damaging.

Your skin also becomes less elastic with age. The lines you form when you move your face may become deeper and more noticeable. Additionally, the collagen and elastin fibers in the dermis become less effective in supporting the skin and keeping it elastic. These natural processes of aging cause the skin to wrinkle and lose its firm texture. Exposure to sunlight accelerates the wrinkling process. Using a sunscreen under your makeup becomes even more important, therefore, as you age.

The goal of a good skin-care program is to minimize the effects of aging on your skin. You can't turn back the clock, but you can take steps to protect your skin against external factors.

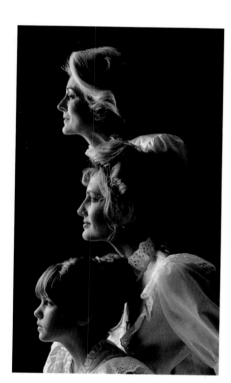

You're never too young — or too old — to practice a program of daily skin care. By taking good care of your skin you can help minimize the effects of aging.

Hormonal Influences Starting at puberty, changing hormone levels contribute to the hyperactivity of the oil glands and may lead to the formation of acne. During your adult life, hormonal levels may also fluctuate to a greater or lesser degree, usually in correspondence with your menstrual cycle and pregnancy.

Various hormones are released throughout your twenty-eight-day menstrual cycle. Some of these hormones stimulate the oil glands, which produce a greater amount of sebum just prior to a menstrual period (and often during and following menstruation). The greater amount of oil production can sometimes be associated with pimples and breakouts (see pages 48 and 49). In addition, research indicates that certain oral contraceptives (particularly the mini-pill and those containing high amounts of synthetic progestins called androgen-dominant pills) contribute to oiliness of the skin and acne formation. These situations can call for a change in your skin-care routine at different points in your menstrual cycle. Using a mask and freshener more frequently may be helpful in controlling excess oil on the skin (see pages 60 to 63).

If your skin is dry, you may be less apt to be affected by hormonal fluctuations during the menstrual cycle. Even dry skin, however, may break out before and during menstruation. If this occurs, you may want to reduce your use of moisturizer and/or night cream during that part of your cycle.

Pregnancy also changes the hormone levels in your body. Your skin may become either very dry and sensitive or excessively oily during pregnancy. If your skin becomes dry, increase your use of moisturizer and night cream. If your skin becomes oily, use a facial mask and freshener more frequently than usual, and reduce your usage of night cream or moisturizer.

Hormonal changes during pregnancy may also increase the production of melanin in your skin, which can result in a number of usually temporary pigmentary disorders, such as freckles and discoloration of certain skin areas. Dark patches, known as chloasma or mask of pregnancy, sometimes appear on the cheeks, near the mouth, or in the brow area during pregnancy. Irregular pigmentation increases with exposure to the sun; it is recommended that all pregnant women use a highly protective sunscreen (SPF 10 to 15) whenever they are going to be in sunlight.

$\mathcal{S}$pecial Considerations

The top layer of your skin, the epidermis, is your body's single largest and most effective protector from damaging environmental substances. It prevents many toxic materials from getting through your skin's surface and minimizes water loss from deeper tissues. The purpose of regular cleansing is to remove environmental pollution or soils from the *surface* of your skin to make your facial skin look, feel, and function better.

The coating of oil from the sebaceous glands and water from the eccrine sweat glands increases the protective function of the epidermis. In areas where the climate is extremely dry, this coating evaporates so rapidly that it becomes difficult for the oil and sweat glands to replenish lubricants on the facial surface. The use of protective cosmetics — foundations and/or moisturizers — helps hold the important oil and water supplies on the skin's surface.

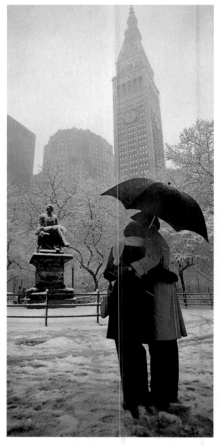

To conserve body heat when the weather is very cold, the blood vessels in the dermis constrict. It is a good idea to keep your face, neck, and ears well covered in winter, to help keep your skin warm. When skin is warm, the blood vessels function more easily by supplying necessary nutrients to the skin. In cold weather, too, moisturizer can help protect against moisture loss.

In very hot weather, the sebaceous and sweat glands become more active, supplying excess oil and water to the skin's surface. In hot, dry climates, much of this extra water evaporates naturally. In hot, humid conditions, too much oil can accumulate on the facial surface, possibly contributing to acne-type breakouts (see page 49).

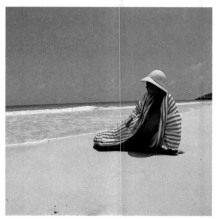

The sun is the environmental factor that is most harmful to the health and appearance of your skin. Ultraviolet radiation — the element of sunlight that most seriously affects the skin — can cause permanent damage if you allow it to penetrate your skin. Ultraviolet rays deteriorate the dermis's collagen and elastin fibers, which enable your skin to retain its elasticity and resist permanent wrinkling. Sun exposure breaks down these substances; the result is skin that sags, loses elasticity, wrinkles, and forms creases. The effects are cumulative. Increasing evidence also links severe sunburn early in life to serious forms of skin cancer later on.

Exposure to the sun does have some benefits. Sun exposure increases the available blood volume that circulates throughout the body, giving us a sense of well-being. It also provides us with vitamin

Sun Tips

For maximum effectiveness, apply a sunscreen seven to fifteen minutes before your skin will be exposed to the sun.

Choose a sunscreen product you can spread evenly in a thick film on your facial skin; thin and uneven applications do not provide sufficient protection.

Apply sunscreen to all the exposed areas of your head, including the part in your hair, the tops of your ears, the top of your brow, your neck, and your neckline. Another sensitive area to remember is the tops of your feet if you wear sandals or go barefoot.

Protection is important no matter how dark your skin is. Even very tan or black skin is vulnerable to ultraviolet radiation.

If you engage in sports that make you perspire, reapply sunscreen regularly to maintain its effectiveness.

Ultraviolet radiation penetrates water, so use your sunscreen when you swim, and reapply it afterward.

Ultraviolet rays penetrate clouds and haze, so use a sunscreen even when the sun isn't shining. And don't feel an umbrella at the beach is sufficient protection. Sand can reflect rays, so you should wear a sunscreen anytime you're at the beach.

Sun damage occurs whenever you are in the sun, not just when you are most conscious of it. Time spent outdoors shopping, gardening, or walking can add up to more sun exposure over a lifetime than time spent at the beach, by a pool, biking, swimming, or boating. Always protect your skin with a sunscreen when you know you will be outdoors.

D for our bones, teeth, and hormonal systems. But weigh the advantages against the disadvantages of sun exposure, and consider that its benefits still exist when you apply a sunscreen. The use of a sunscreen to maintain a smooth and youthful complexion is perhaps the most important element in caring for your skin. A sunscreen with a sun protection factor (SPF) of at least 10 blocks most of the sun's ultraviolet radiation before it can damage your skin. (The SPF number indicates the length of time a given product will protect your skin. Using a sunscreen with an SPF of 10, a person who begins to burn within twenty minutes of exposure to bright noonday sun can tolerate the same kind of sun ten times longer, or almost four hours, before burning.)

Your heredity and the amount of time you spend in the sun can compound the risks and make the use of a sunscreen even more important in protecting the health and appearance of your skin. The danger of sun damage increases if you are fair-haired and/or fair-skinned, or freckle easily; if you live in the Sun Belt; or if your occupation or leisure activities keep you regularly exposed to strong sun. Other significant factors include:

Time of year: exposure to ultraviolet rays reaches its dangerous peak on June 21 in the northern hemisphere, lasting through August; but you need protection as early as April, long before the hottest days of August.

Time of day: the sun's rays are most intense, and thus most dangerous, between 10:00 A.M. and 2:00 P.M. (11:00 A.M. and 3:00 P.M. daylight saving time).

Altitude: at high altitudes, where the atmosphere is thinner, more ultraviolet radiation reaches your skin. You need protection whether you're working or vacationing in mountain regions.

Latitude: the closer you travel to the equator, the greater the amount of ultraviolet radiation. Exposure to ultraviolet radiation — and its concomitant risks — is twice as great in Dallas as in Chicago, for example.

Cumulative and permanent damage from sun exposure can be avoided by using an effective sunscreen. Keep the tips at left in mind. And make protection a natural part of your health-and-beauty-care regimen. It takes just a few minutes, and you'll be glad you didn't neglect it.

Special Considerations

Many of the milder problems you may encounter on your facial skin are caused by extremes in skin type — overly dry or overly oily, for example — and can often be improved with proper skin care. Some problems, however, require specialized care or professional treatment.

Allergies tend to be different in different people. Your way of life — what you eat, where you live, prescription drugs you take — can increase or diminish your allergies. If you notice an allergic reaction — a rash and/or swelling of the skin — and suspect any cleansing or cosmetic product you use on your skin, stop using the product immediately. Take its list of ingredients to a dermatologist or allergist who can help you identify which ingredient is causing the problem and suggest possible alternative products for you to use.

If you use cosmetic preparations *in combination* and develop an allergic response, try a ruling-out procedure. Use no cosmetics at all and observe your skin for one to five days. If the allergic reaction improves dramatically or disappears within this period, you may assume that it was associated with one of the products you used. Next, use a small amount of one product at a time for a minimum of five days, carefully observing your skin's reaction to it. If a strong reaction occurs, discontinue using that product. When you discover which product caused the allergy, seek a dermatologist's or allergist's aid if you wish to be patch-tested for individual ingredients.

Two other common skin disorders are *seborrheic dermatitis* and *rosacea*. Seborrheic dermatitis results from the excessive secretion of sebum and produces scaling and itching of the facial skin, most often in the areas of the eyebrow, along the edges of the nose, and behind the ears. It can easily be mistaken for dryness, but unlike common dry skin, this condition does not improve when a moisturizer is used. Rosacea is a face rash that produces redness and pimples in adults, especially on the nose, mid-forehead, chin, and cheeks. Causes of the rash are unknown, but it has been found that in some cases the condition is aggravated by the ingestion of alcoholic beverages, spicy foods, coffee, or tea. A dermatologist can diagnose and treat these conditions.

Lack of melanin in a specific area of the skin may produce white patches, a condition called *vitiligo*. Conversely, excessive pigmentation on certain parts of the skin surface produces dark areas; *birth-*

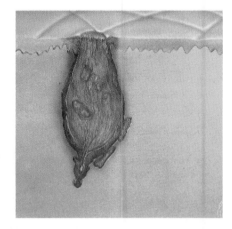

Surface irregularities on the skin begin below its surface. When the hair follicle fills with dead skin cells, bacteria, and oils, it can lead to an open comedo, or blackhead, as illustrated here, or to a pimple. Good skin care can help prevent unsightly breakouts.

Acne: A Common Skin Condition

While acne is generally associated with puberty, this condition can also appear for the first time in adults in their twenties or thirties. At any age, heredity, drugs, or oily cosmetics can add excess oil to skin already over-supplied with sebum. Other causes may include comedogenic (pore-clogging) chemicals, stress, heat, and humidity.

Acne was once thought to be caused by certain foods, dirty skin, or unapproved behaviors. Today, acne is believed to be associated with overly oily skin and genetic and psychological factors, such as stress. The latest acne research reports that it is probably a result of a buildup of keratin proteins, bacteria, and oils in the ducts (exits) of some hair follicles; large follicles located on the face, chest, and upper back are most susceptible.

In teenagers, rapidly rising hormone levels cause the sebaceous (oil) glands to enlarge and produce more oil. These same hormones can cause excess keratin to plug follicle openings, resulting in the most basic type of acne lesion, the *comedo*.

Comedones are composed of bacteria trapped in the hair follicles and overly active keratin cells. Normally, skin cells shed while they are in the process of moving up to the epidermis; comedones form when the cells aren't shed, filling up the follicles. Some comedones may develop into the typical inflamed acne lesions.

Pimples and pustules can develop from comedones when the walls of the plugged follicles rupture, spreading the dead skin cells, oil, and bacteria into the dermis. The blood vessels below the skin then become enlarged to accommodate more white blood cells, which are needed to combat the infection in the lower layers of the skin. The enlarged blood vessels cause the skin to appear red, and the white blood cells combine with the dead skin cells, sebum, and bacteria impacted in the follicle to form pus. The result is a red pimple with a yellowish head, called a pustule, which forms on the surface of the skin.

Once the pimple has formed, it is unwise to squeeze out the material trapped there; at worst, it forces bacteria deeper into the skin and can cause scarring. If pustules form on your face, chest, and/or back, consult a dermatologist.

If your skin is prone to acne-type breakouts, keep it clean so that excess sebum, bacteria, and dead skin cells on the skin's surface do not contribute to pore blockage. However, once acne is present, excessive scrubbing or frequent cleansing will not control it, and any rough manipulation of the skin may further irritate and inflame the lesions. Diet is no longer considered to be significant as a cause of acne in most individuals. However, if you suspect a particular food as the cause of an occasional pimple, remove that food from your diet for a few weeks and observe your skin to see if its condition improves.

Medical research has developed a variety of ways to treat differing stages and degrees of acne. If you suspect you have incipient acne or the condition is apparent on your skin, consult a dermatologist as soon as possible.

Skin Care

marks are a form of hyperpigmentation. If such pigmentary disorders disturb you, seek medical advice.

Another common form of hyperpigmentation is *facial moles*. These usually harmless spots sometimes sprout hair. As you age the moles tend to lighten and become more raised. However, if you notice an obvious change in a mole or if one begins to bleed, consult a dermatologist immediately.

Cold sores and *fever blisters* are caused by a form of the herpes virus, for which there is currently no known cure. Vaccines are now being tested and may be available within a few years. The virus remains in the skin where it first erupted and can be aggravated to run its course again by sunburn, scratching, or stress.

Facial warts, which are also caused by a virus, can be removed. Your dermatologist can advise you concerning treatment.

Taking a Closer Look

The type of skin you have determines how you should care for it. The following questionnaire will help you identify your apparent skin type and the kind of skin-care routine you should follow. Keep in mind that this inventory can give you only a very general classification of the condition of your skin. It may change with age as well as with the seasons. You are also likely to observe improvements once you've established a proper program for skin care.

Mark the boxes below that best describe the way your skin looks and feels at this point in your life. Then look at the skin type listed beneath the column in which you marked the most boxes; this is your skin type at this time. As your skin changes, you will want to take this inventory again; it's best to review your answers about four times a year, at the beginning of each season. Your answers may also depend on the type of products you have recently been using to care for your skin.

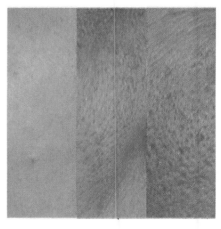

Magnified views (from left to right) of small, medium, and large pores.

1. Six hours after cleansing, my skin usually feels:

☐ Very dry to moderately dry

☐ Relatively unchanged: well-lubricated but not oily or dry

☐ Oily on my forehead, nose, and chin (the T-zone), drier on cheeks and sides of face

☐ Very oily

2. Three hours after applying a typical liquid foundation (one not formulated for any specific skin type), my facial surface appears:

☐ Matte (dull) in finish, with no shine

☐ Soft and smooth, neither dull nor shiny

☐ Somewhat shiny in my T-zone

☐ Very shiny

3. Whiteheads, blackheads, and small bumps appear on my facial skin:

☐ Almost never

☐ Very rarely, possibly before and/or during menstruation

☐ Sometimes, especially on my forehead or chin or near my nose

☐ Almost always

4. The small lines that form on my face with facial movements tend to remain "imprinted" on my skin:

☐ Around my mouth and eyes and on my forehead

☐ Very faintly near my eyes, and increasingly as I get older

☐ Just around my eyes, and possibly near my mouth

☐ For a short time, then they disappear

5. My facial pores are:

☐ So small they can barely be seen

☐ Small to medium and regular in size over the surface of my whole face

☐ Medium to large; noticeably larger in my T-zone

☐ Large, especially in my T-zone and on my cheeks

6. As compared to five years ago, my facial skin has become:

☐ Quite a bit drier

☐ Slightly drier

☐ Drier only on the sides of my cheeks and the outside edges of my face

☐ Not noticeably drier; possibly more oily

DRY   NORMAL   COMBINATION   OILY

7. Regardless of the products I use, my skin feels tight and dry:

☐ Often

☐ Occasionally in extremely cold or dry weather

☐ Only on the sides of my cheeks and the outside edges of my face

☐ Rarely or never

8. Some areas of my face tend to become oily:

☐ Rarely

☐ Occasionally, in extremely hot or humid weather

☐ Usually in my T-zone

☐ Almost always

9. My skin tends to chap:

☐ Frequently, on both my hands and face

☐ Occasionally, on both my hands and face, when exposed to extremely dry or cold weather

☐ Only on the sides of my cheeks and the outside edges of my face; possibly on my hands

☐ Rarely or never on my face; sometimes on my hands, in extremely dry or cold weather

| **DRY** | **NORMAL** | **COMBINATION** | **OILY** |

Your Skin Type

Record your skin type and the date you have taken this inventory in the space provided below. Look for special considerations for your skin type throughout this book to help establish the best skin-care and beauty program for yourself. If you change your diet, or you find yourself in a dramatically different climate, or you start or stop taking medication, review this inventory again a few weeks after such a change. Each time you take the inventory, note the changes and improvements in your skin so you can make appropriate adjustments in your beauty routine.

Date	Skin type	Remarks

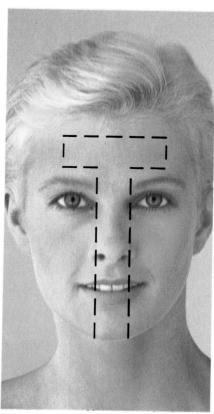

The T-zone

$\mathcal{D}$iscovering Your Skin Type

No one has skin exactly like anyone else. In order for your skin-care program to work effectively, your routine must be designed to meet the individual needs of *your* skin. There are basically four types of skin — dry, normal, combination, and oily. The personal inventory of skin type on pages 50 and 51 can help you determine which category describes your own skin.

Dry skin is usually characterized by small pores and a matte (dull) finish, with little or no superficial shine. Expression lines form readily on dry skin, first on the brow, then around the eyes and near the lips. Dry skin is most typical in women over the age of thirty-five and those who live in either hot or cold low-humidity climates. Dry skin may also develop among women who spend a great deal of time outdoors without properly protecting their skin from the elements. Such skin becomes rough and may flake or crack.

Because environmental factors dry the surface of your face without actually affecting the deeper sebaceous glands that produce and secrete your skin's oils, it is sometimes difficult to determine whether you really have dry skin. Our personal inventory of skin type helps you explore the nature of your skin in a way that will enable you to recognize your skin's true type and adjust your skin-care program accordingly.

Normal skin has a smooth texture and, at best, a fine, porcelain-like quality. Lines and wrinkles seldom form on this type of skin until rather late in life. Normal skin rarely, if ever, develops white-heads, blackheads, or pimples.

Although many women may describe their skin as normal, it is actually a rather rare type. If you are lucky enough to have been born with normal skin (for, in fact, heredity is a major factor behind skin type), you need a good program of care to maintain its excellent condition.

Combination skin is probably the most common skin type among women in their twenties and thirties. It is characterized by moderate to very oily conditions in the T-zone (the area forming a T across the forehead and down the center of the face, running down the nose and onto the chin), combined with variably dry skin at the outside edges of the face — cheeks, temples, outer corners of the eyes, jawline, and possibly the areas surrounding the upper lip and the corners of the mouth.

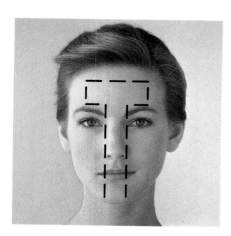

The T-zone

The appearance of combination skin varies from a shiny and large-pored texture in the T-zone to smaller pores and a more matte finish of the outer edges of the face. This type of skin can be cared for with a regular and healthful skin-care program that controls oil in oily areas and adds moisture to drier areas.

Oily skin results when the sebaceous glands produce too much oil, giving skin a shiny appearance, and sometimes a greasy or sticky feel. Oily skin tends to wrinkle less readily than drier skin types. The large amount of oil on the skin's surface may help the upper layers hold onto water and protects the skin from environmental causes of dryness. However, this skin type is prone to acne-type breakouts well beyond adolescence. Good skin care can help control excess oiliness and the formation of whiteheads, blackheads, and pimples. Oily skin usually has larger pores than other skin types. Use of the proper skin-care products and procedures helps make the pores appear smaller and the face smoother and less shiny.

Although you can't change your skin type, you can change the condition of your skin with proper care and adequate protection. After completing your personal inventory of skin type, you will be able to note special considerations and recommendations for your skin type throughout the five steps to beautiful skin, which follow. Knowing your skin type allows you to personalize your skin-care routine and to take that first step toward your own special beauty.

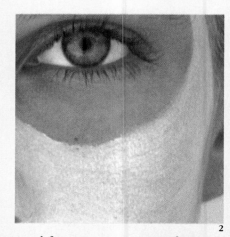

5 steps to Beautiful Skin

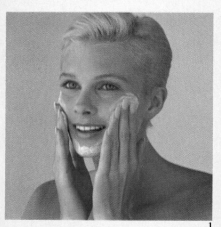

Your skin is the translucent background for your expressive features and for the glamorous makeup you apply. A careful program of skin care soon results in skin that is smooth, soft, and glowing — skin that displays the pride you take in yourself and your desire to look and feel your best. A clear, radiant complexion may sometimes seem hard to achieve, but it is attainable by everyone, and it is the first and most important step to a woman's total beauty.

The five steps to beautiful skin — cleanse, stimulate, freshen, moisturize, and protect — form a beauty-care program based on scientific research about what is best for your skin. Each of the steps has a scientific basis related to the many roles your skin plays every day. For your skin-care program to work effectively, it is important that you use all five steps. Each step is simple to perform, and together they can become a very pleasant and relaxing part of your daily beauty routine.

The five steps to beautiful skin work well for each of the four different skin types — dry, normal, combination, and oily. While no skin-care program can change your skin type, the five steps to beautiful skin can improve the condition of your skin and accentuate its most positive elements.

In the pages that follow, you will learn the scientific importance of each step, how to choose appropriate products for your specific skin type, and how and when to apply them. Everything you need and want to know about your personal skin-care program is right here at your fingertips. You'll soon want to make the five steps to beautiful skin a part of your daily beauty routine.

1 *Cleanse*

Clean, soft skin with a fresh and dewy luster can be achieved only by consistent, careful cleansing. Creams and cleansers soften your skin while they gently loosen and remove the soils that can dull the surface of your face.

2 *Stimulate*

A refreshing facial mask increases the blood circulation that brings healthful nourishment to the skin.

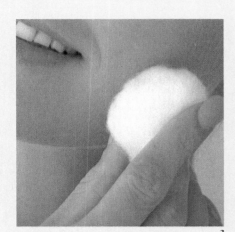

3

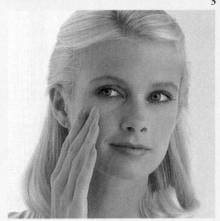

4

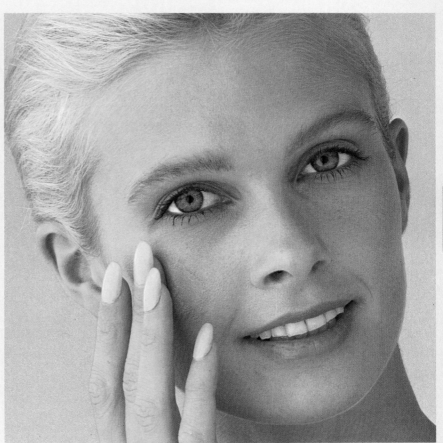

5

3 *Freshen*
A freshener stimulates and tones
the surface of your facial skin, and
removes the last traces of your
cleanser or mask. This toning function helps restore the proper acid
balance of your skin.

4 *Moisturize*
A moisturizer softens and conditions your skin, endowing it with a
youthful softness and a lustrous
patina, added suppleness and
elasticity.

5 *Protect*
A sunscreen and makeup foundation shields your face from direct
contact with dirt or pollutants in
the air, and helps prevent your skin
from losing its necessary moisture.
Foundation also adds a hint of
subtle color and an even-toned
texture to your face. Sunscreen
shields your skin against the damaging ultraviolet rays and helps re-
tard the aging effects of exposure
to the sun.

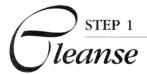

Cleanse

Your skin is exposed to many elements every day. Cleansing removes the substances that can accumulate on your face — makeup, excess sebum (oil), dirt and pollutants, and dead skin cells. These substances may contribute to pore-clogging and keep the top layer of skin from functioning efficiently.

Dry skin seems to produce a minimal amount of natural oil and water for lubricating the skin, so a cleanser for dry skin must be able to remove both superficial impurities and dry, flaking skin cells *without* removing the necessary oil and moisture on the skin's surface. A rich, highly emollient cleansing cream, dense in texture and high in oil content, is best for dry skin.

Normal and combination skin require the same cleansing treatment. It must loosen and remove cosmetics and surface soils, lift off dead skin cells, and clear away excess oil, particularly in the T-zone area of the face.

An effective cleanser for both these skin types should cleanse the face and pick up extra oils where they have accumulated; at the same time it shouldn't dry other, less oily parts of the face. A light, fluffy, water-soluble cleansing cream that can be easily removed with a damp facecloth is the best formula for these two skin types.

Oily skin requires special cleansing because the excess sebum that coats the facial surface may tend to trap dead skin cells. In addition, soils adhere more readily to oily skin and may be more difficult to remove. The best cleanser for oily skin is one that effectively loosens and removes surface soils, dead skin cells, and a larger amount of excess oil without stripping away the skin's natural moisture. A foaming, liquid cleanser that produces a sudsy lather with water is the best formula for oily skin.

Whatever your skin type, a daily cleansing routine is a must. It's also important to cleanse in the proper manner, using a special technique that we'll describe on pages 58 and 59.

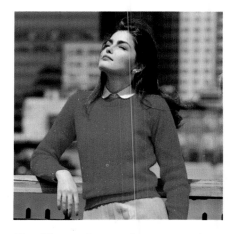

City life can be tough on your skin; air pollution and other environmental soils may interfere with your skin's functions. A daily cleansing routine helps counteract the potential damage of an urban environment.

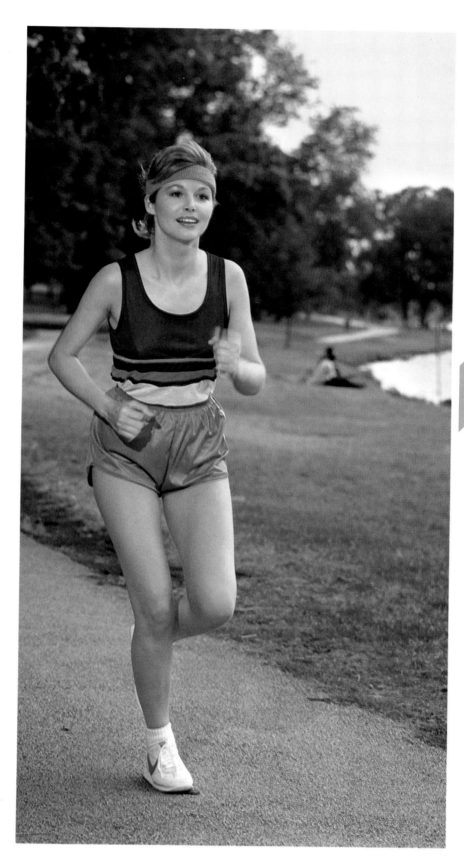

Glowing good looks are within
your reach — and they start with
an ongoing skin-care routine. Step
number one: cleansing, to help
keep skin clear and fresh.

57

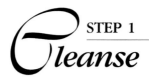 Cleanse

When you use any cleansing product, apply it gently to avoid pulling the delicate surface of your face. Begin by putting the cleanser on your fingertips. Starting at the base of your neck, lightly stroke upward and outward, on to your neck and up over your chin and jawline, as shown in the photo at right. Then, still using your fingertips, move upward over the area surrounding your mouth and on to the sides of your cheeks and temples. Next, work the cleanser upward and outward over your forehead, just above the eyebrows, and upward to the hairline. Then stroke it down the bridge and sides of your nose (the *only* area on which downward movements are used). When you apply any product near your eyes, always use your ring finger as it exerts the least pressure in an area where the facial skin is thinnest and most delicate. Below your eyes, stroke gently inward from the outside of your eyes toward the bridge of your nose. Never scrub or harshly manipulate any area of your face, as all pulling and tugging of your skin can damage its fragile tissues and contribute to wrinkling.

Dry, normal, and combination skin should be cleansed in the manner described above. Apply the recommended products with light strokes of the fingers. Next, dampen a facecloth with warm water, and using the same movement of application, gently yet thoroughly remove the cleansing cream with the cloth.

Oily skin should be cleansed with a foaming product. Shake the cleanser before spreading it on your neck and face, using the application described above. Next, lightly pat water on top of the cleanser and, with light upward and outward strokes, work the cleanser into a foam. Then splash your skin with warm water and remove all traces of the cleanser with a warm, wet facecloth.

When to Cleanse Whatever your skin type, you should cleanse your face thoroughly every evening to remove the day's accumulation of makeup, dirt, and oil. Always be sure to remove any residue of the cleanser at the sides of your mouth, in the crevices near your nostrils, and along your hairline. If your skin is oily, you might also want to cleanse in the morning to remove the excess oil secreted and accumulated on your skin overnight. Otherwise, you can start the day by simply freshening your skin (see pages 62 and 63). Cleansing begins the skin-softening process and leaves your skin beautifully smooth — and ready for the skin-care steps to follow.

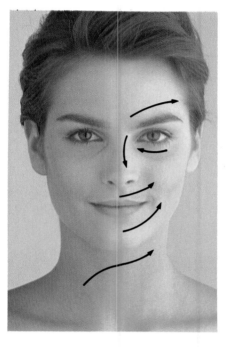

The right movement of application is important in every step of your skin-care program. Always avoid pulling, tugging, or stressing the delicate surface of your skin.

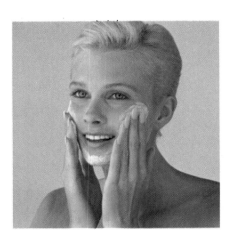

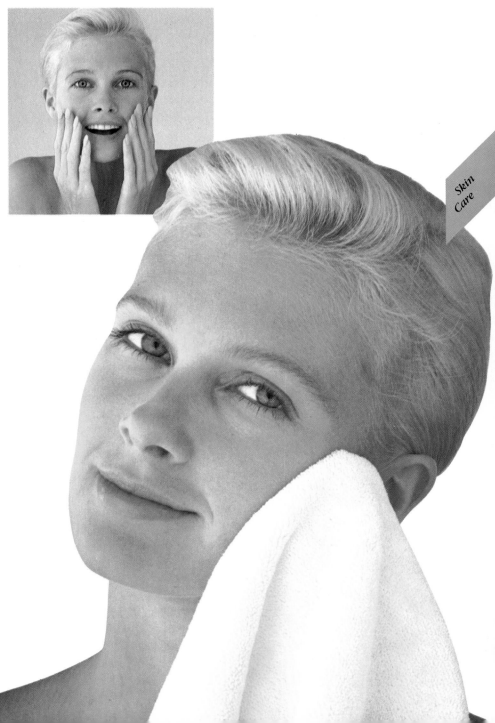

Cleansing feels great — and gives your skin a healthy glow. For the fresh feeling of properly cleansed skin, apply the cleanser recommended for your skin type, using the movement of application shown at left. Next, dampen a facecloth with warm water and remove the cleanser gently and thoroughly. Make the most of this important step in your personal beauty routine; you'll see and feel the healthy benefits. Cleansing is the first essential step in your daily skincare routine.

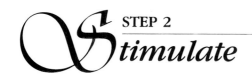

Stimulate

Because the cells on the top layer of your skin are continually being replaced, dead cells can accumulate and may cause a slowdown in normal epidermal functions. Regular use of a facial mask removes these dead cells. It also makes your pores appear smaller, and stimulates the circulation of blood in your face, bringing oxygen and other essential nutrients to the skin. When used regularly and in conjunction with the other steps to beautiful skin, a facial mask can give your complexion a magical luster.

Dry and normal skin need the frequent use of a mask to remove dead skin cells. A mask for these skin types should contain a mild abrasive to remove dead skin cells. It should also have a creamy texture that does not strip oil and moisture from the skin's surface.

Combination and oily skin require similar formulas in a mask. Where excess sebum is present, dead cells can become trapped in oily sheets on the skin's surface. A mask helps remove the excess oils and accumulated dead skin cells. The oilier your skin, the more you need a highly oil-absorbent mask to remove the excess sebum. Clay-based masks, which dry and harden on the skin's surface, pick up oil. Choosing a mask for combination skin depends on your skin's special characteristics: if your skin tends to be dry, use a cream-based moisturizing mask; for oilier skin, use a clay-based mask.

How and When to Stimulate Whatever your skin type, you should apply your facial mask the way that's pictured at the right. If you have dry skin, it is especially important that you use featherlike movements of your fingers and avoid massaging the mask onto your skin.

Also regardless of your skin type, you should mask twice a week at regular intervals in the evening after cleansing. If your skin is very oily, or if it tends to be excessively oily in hot or more humid conditions, you may have to use a facial mask more often, perhaps as frequently as every other day.

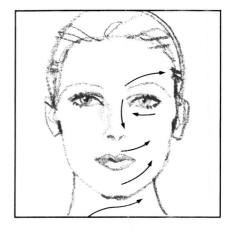

Proper movement of application

The stimulation of a mask does wonders for the condition of your skin. This second step is relaxing and beautifying; it leaves your skin feeling refreshed, vibrant, and alive. Apply the facial mask recommended for your skin type with featherlike strokes in the manner shown above; avoid the delicate areas around your eyes and mouth. Allow the mask to dry (approximately ten minutes), then place a warm, wet facecloth over your mask to soften it for removal. Wipe off the mask gently, using the recommended movement of application. For best results, mask at least twice a week.

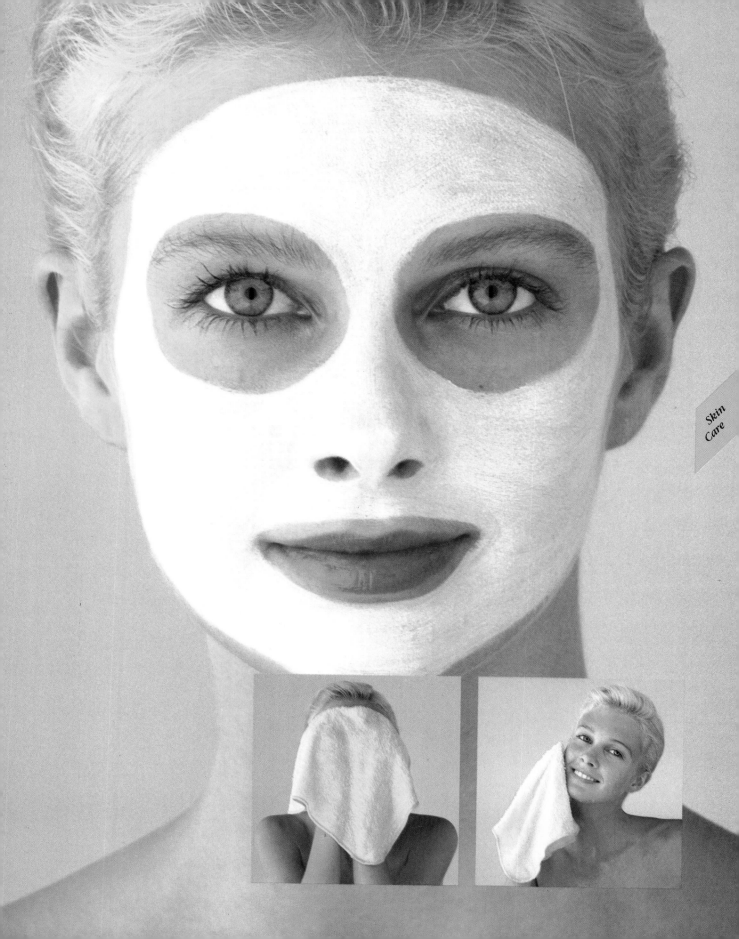

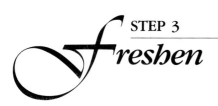

Freshen

Skin freshener does just what its name implies: it freshens the skin by removing any remaining surface impurities as well as any residue of your cleanser or mask. A skin freshener may also be referred to as an astringent, toner, tonique, or refining or texture lotion. It restores the protective acid balance of the skin, improves circulation and oxygen exchange in the skin, and helps pores appear smaller.

Dry and normal skin both require a freshener that cleans off all traces of cleansers, masks, and soils without making the skin parched and taut. A liquid freshener, which tingles somewhat when applied (but does not burn), is best for dry skin.

Combination and oily skin both require a liquid freshener that leaves the skin feeling refreshed and clean, not tight and dry. Oily skin especially responds to a liquid freshener that "degreases" the skin's surface, reducing shine on the face. A freshener can make larger pores associated with oily skin appear smaller.

How and When to Freshen When applying a freshener as shown in the diagram at right, you may experience a mild tingling sensation. If you have dry skin, you can counteract this sensation by moistening a cotton pad with tepid water before putting the freshener on it. If you have combination skin, which is very oily in some areas and very dry in others, moisten the cotton pad with warm water before applying the freshener to those areas of your face that are especially dry. Apply the freshener full strength on oilier areas. If your skin is especially oily, or if soils and residues seem to cling to your face, you may want to apply freshener a second time.

Use a freshener twice a day, every day. It is your first step in the morning and your second step in the evening (unless you choose to mask first on a particular day), after cleansing.

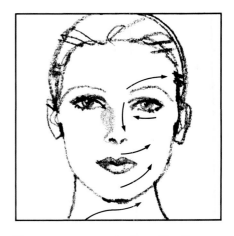

Proper movement of application

Luxuriate in the smooth, even texture of skin freshened daily. This important step refines your pores, further stimulates circulation, and removes the residue of any previously used product. Moisten a cotton ball with a few drops of the freshener for your skin type. Apply it with gentle upward and outward strokes, avoiding the delicate areas around your eyes and mouth, as shown at right. Allow the freshener to dry naturally. Your skin will immediately look brighter, feel fresher.

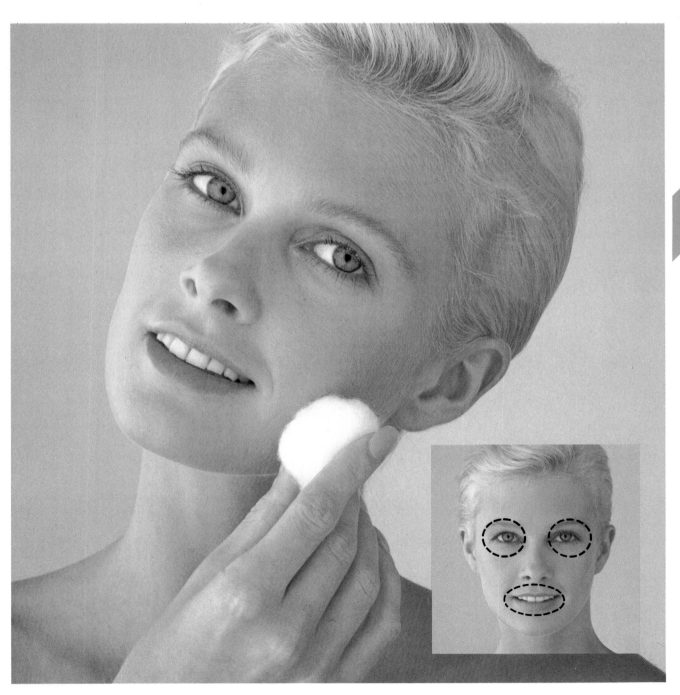

Moisturize

Your face is constantly exposed to environments that cause important moisture — the moisture that keeps your skin soft and fresh-looking — to evaporate. Moisturizer helps the top layer of your skin retain its natural water content by providing ingredients that attract water and seal it into the top layers of the skin. Moisturizer conditions the texture of your skin, thereby minimizing the appearance of lines and small wrinkles that form where skin is driest. *All* types of skin need some type of moisturizing.

Dry skin loses water from its facial surface more rapidly than other types of skin. If you have dry skin, use both a night cream and a daytime moisturizer. A night cream lubricates your facial skin and replenishes the oil your skin needs. A light, liquid daytime moisturizer provides a soft, smoother surface for the application of makeup while helping to retain the skin's essential moisture.

Normal and combination skin need moisturizers to maintain the natural moisture content of the facial surface and to replenish oils in dry areas. Both skin types require a night cream that is light in texture and does not leave a greasy feel or a shiny look. During the day, apply a light lotion moisturizer to soften and condition dry areas.

Oily skin needs minimal moisturizing because its sebum may help seal in the water. Nonetheless, even oily skin may require some moisturization in dry areas — around your eyes, the sides of your cheeks, and your neck. If you have oily skin, apply a light and gentle moisturizer, either at night or during the day, only on those areas that feel and appear to be dry.

How and When to Moisturize Dry skin should be moisturized at night after cleansing, masking (on appropriate days), and freshening. Moisten your face and neck with warm water. Then gently apply a small amount of night cream to your skin, following the proper movement of application as indicated in the diagram at right. With light strokes of your fingertips, smooth the night cream on your skin until it seems to disappear, and leave it on overnight.

Apply daytime moisturizer after freshening with light upward and outward movements. If you have very *dry skin*, use a daytime moisturizer under your foundation; if your skin is dry only in certain areas — around your eyes, near your mouth, at the sides of your

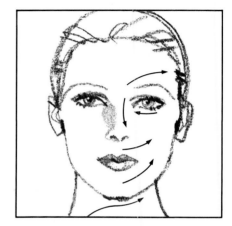

Proper movement of application

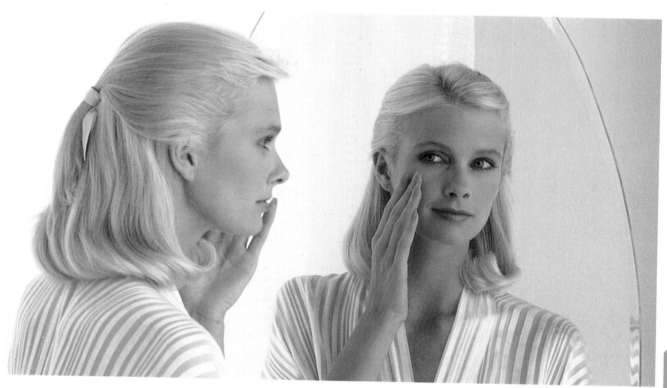

cheeks — moisturize only those areas before applying foundation. (Remember to use your ring finger in gentle patting movements when applying moisturizer near your eyes.)

Normal and combination skin need the nighttime moisturization of a light cream applied in very small amounts after cleansing, masking (on appropriate days), and freshening. Smooth the moisturizer over your neck and face with gentle upward and outward movements of the fingertips, as indicated in the diagram at left. During the day, both types of skin should be moisturized (after freshening), but sparingly and only in those areas that appear dehydrated. Use your ring finger to pat the moisturizer gently on the skin near your eyes.

Oily skin should be moisturized after using freshener only in those areas of your neck or face that look and feel dry. In the eye area, use your ring finger to apply moisturizer to the skin. Oily skin requires moisturization in the evening on the dry areas only. Apply the moisturizer after cleansing, masking (on appropriate days), and freshening. In the morning after cleansing and freshening, apply moisturizer only to those areas of skin that appear to be dehydrated.

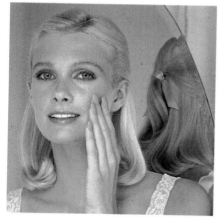

Almost every type of skin needs moisturizer — whether you apply it in the morning only or morning and evening. It soothes, lubricates, and conditions your skin, helping conceal the fine lines that form on dry skin and retain precious moisture in dry areas on oily skin.

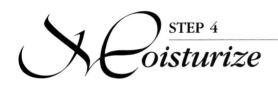
Moisturize

Your skin's moisturizing needs may vary with changes in the seasons or with travel from one climate to another. Generally, heat causes your skin's oil glands to become more active. When weather is also humid, oil and water cannot evaporate naturally, so oils remain on the skin, coating the facial surface.

In hot and dry weather, the heat may stimulate excess oil production. But water tends to evaporate from the skin's surface in a dry atmosphere, so overoiliness is not such a great problem. Dry skin, however, can suffer in this climate because hot, dry air can lead to extreme dehydration. When you are exposed to the sun daily, your skin requires protection from its rays (see pages 46 and 47 and 68 and 69).

In cold and dry conditions, your oil production may become sluggish, limiting the supply of oil to your skin. These conditions can cause your skin to chap, especially in cold, windy weather.

Humid air is beneficial to most skin types because it helps facial skin hold onto its moisture content. However, cold and damp conditions can affect dry skin problems; hot and damp conditions can affect oily skin problems.

Both the cool, dry environment of air conditioning and the hot, dry conditions of artificial heating can dry your skin. In addition, since indoor cooling and heating systems counteract the outdoor climate, your skin may react erratically after being subjected to widely varying conditions. You must take all these changes into account when you use the chart at right. If you live in a hot, humid climate, but spend most of your time in an air-conditioned office and house, you should follow the moisturizing suggestions for a cold, dry environment. Similarly, if you live in a cold and damp area but are usually indoors in heated rooms, you should follow the suggestions for a hot, dry environment.

The chart offers guidelines on moisturizing your skin, but you should also use your own senses of sight and touch to note your skin's reactions. Whenever your skin feels greasier and looks shinier than usual, cut down or eliminate moisturizing, and possibly use a mask more often. When your skin feels tight and appears to be parched, increase your use of moisturizer.

Using Moisturizer in Different Climates

Skin Type	Environment			
	Hot and Humid	Cold and Dry	Hot and Dry	Cold and Damp
Dry	Use a rich night cream to help hold oil and moisture on your skin's surface. You may need a daytime moisturizer only for your neck and the dehydrated areas of your face—around your eyes.	It's very important to use a rich night cream every night, as well as a moisturizer under your foundation (see pages 70 to 75) every day.	Use a rich night cream every night and a daytime moisturizer daily.	Use a rich night cream every night and a daytime moisturizer as needed, especially in cold, windy weather.
Normal	Use a light night cream to help your skin hold its natural oil and water content.	Use a light night cream every night to seal in water. You may need to apply a daytime moisturizer on the drier areas of your face. In cold, windy conditions, apply moisturizer to your entire face and neck.	Use a light night cream and a daytime moisturizer where needed on drier facial areas, such as the skin surrounding your eyes and mouth, and on your neck.	Use a light night cream and a daytime moisturizer where needed: on your neck and near your eyes. In cold, windy weather, use a daytime moisturizer on your entire face and neck.
Combina-tion	Avoid applying any moisturizer to your T-zone area, and use a daytime moisturizer only *if needed* on the drier areas—your neck, the sides of your cheeks, and the outer edges of your face.	Use a daytime moisturizer on your neck, the sides of your cheeks, and the outer edges of your face. If this skin becomes especially dry, use a light night cream as well.	Avoid applying any moisturizer to your T-zone area, and use a daytime moisturizer on drier areas—your neck, the sides of your cheeks, and the outer edges of your face.	As needed, use a daytime moisturizer on your neck, the sides of your cheeks, and the outer edges of your face.
Oily	Use no moisturizer except on very dry areas—possibly around your eyes and lips. Mask more frequently.	Use a daytime moisturizer on the drier areas near your eyes and possibly on your neck.	Use a daytime moisturizer sparingly on drier areas, near your eyes and on your neck, if needed.	Use a daytime moisturizer on the drier areas of your face, around your eyes, and on your neck, if needed.

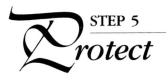rotect

The final step in your five steps to beautiful skin is the essential protect step — the application of foundation and, when needed, sunscreen. A foundation helps protect your skin from dehydrating conditions and pollutants in the environment; it covers small imperfections on your facial surface and gives your complexion an even-toned finish. Properly applied foundation also evens out skin pigmentation and adds a subtle glow of color.

For extra protection from the sun's harmful ultraviolet rays, add a facial under-makeup sunscreen to your skin-care routine. Apply sunscreen before your foundation; if your skin is dry, apply sunscreen over your daytime moisturizer. If you use a moisturizer only on dehydrated areas, apply your moisturizer first, before your sunscreen and foundation.

Dry skin benefits from a creamy, oil-based foundation that helps form a seal to lock in moisture and adds extra lubrication to the skin, thereby minimizing the fine lines typical of drier skin. In addition, drier skin may be thinner, allowing veins and dark areas under the eyes to appear. You can cover them with a concealing foundation (see page 73).

Normal skin also needs a creamy, oil-based foundation that helps seal in the skin's natural moisture and protects it from environmental soils and dehydration. The foundation should give the skin a soft, natural sheen without shine.

Combination and oily skin need a water-based liquid foundation that absorbs surface oils and reduces shine without drying the skin. The irregular and larger pores characteristic of both these skin types can be improved by foundations that make the skin's surface appear smoother and more regular. If your skin tends to develop blemishes, you may want to use special application techniques to minimize facial imperfections (see page 73).

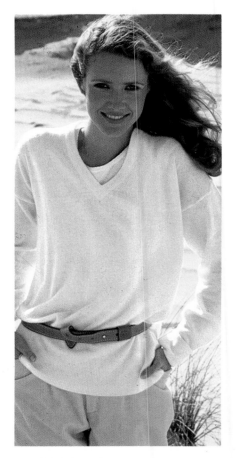

Youthful, healthy-looking skin demands daily protection. Because the sun, more than any other single factor, can damage your skin, you'll want to make sure always to use a sunscreen outdoors.

Using Sunscreen

Use of a sunscreen is an important element in your daily skin-care program *whenever* you are going to be exposed to sunlight. Remember that even in city settings and in the winter your skin absorbs ultraviolet radiation from the sun. If you live in a high altitude, or in an urban location where many buildings have glass or other reflective surfaces, you may have to use a sunscreen every day. Given all that is known about the damaging effects of sunlight on the skin, the best rule to keep in mind is: when in doubt, *use* a sunscreen.

Cream and lotion sunscreen formulas contain ingredients — the most common are forms of PABA — that provide a physical and/or chemical barrier to the sun's harmful ultraviolet rays. The amount of these barrier in-gredients in a sunscreen determines the product's "sun protection factor," or SPF. This factor is indicated on the container of each product by an SPF number, which may range from 2 to 15. The higher its number, the greater a sunscreen's capacity to protect your skin from damaging ultraviolet radiation.

All types of skin, no matter how dark, require some degree of protection from the sun. Contrary to one popular misconception, sunscreens do not prevent tanning; rather, they reduce tanning and the unwanted effects of sunlight. Sunburn should always be avoided, and when used properly, sunscreens *do* prevent sunburn. To determine the right SPF number for the sunscreen product you should choose, refer to the chart below.

Skin's Usual Reaction to Sun*	Recommended SPF Number
Always burns easily; never tans	10 to 15
Always burns easily; tans minimally	8 to 10
Burns moderately; tans gradually to light brown	6 to 8
Burns minimally; always tans easily to moderate brown	4 to 6
Rarely burns; tans quickly to dark brown	2 to 4

* Based on the first thirty to forty-five minutes of exposure to the sun after a winter season of no such exposure.

Skin Tones: Nature's Palette

A foundation — the final step in your basic skin-care program — not only protects your skin, it also provides the base for all your glamour cosmetics. The first step in selecting your foundation is determining what you want your makeup base to do. Studies show that the majority of women want a foundation that matches their natural color; the shade you choose should be as close to your skin tone as possible to blend and even out your facial colors. At other times, however, you may prefer your skin to have a bright, sun-kissed appearance. In addition, you may want to conceal minor imperfections with foundation.

The women pictured here illustrate the wide spectrum of skin tones. Their selection of foundation was

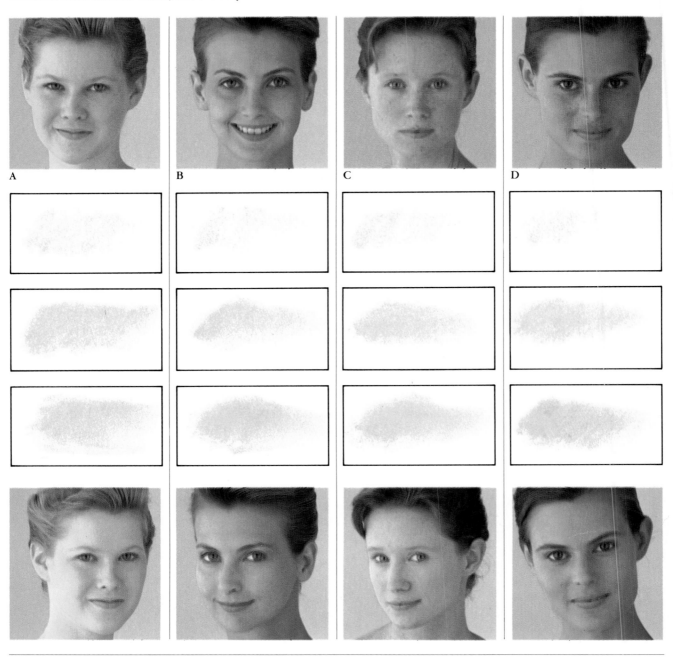

A   B   C   D

based on a scientific measurement of their skin color. In the top photographs the women's faces are clean; in the bottom photographs, each woman is wearing the foundation shade that comes closest to her natural tone. The color swatches show other complementary foundation shade possibilities. These alternatives can help you attain a range of looks — from covering freckles to making your complexion appear beautifully bronzed.

How do you know what shades will work for you?

Because it is unlikely you will ever have your skin color measured scientifically, it is always best to try before you buy. Test foundations on your face in natural lighting. The inventory on the following pages will help you determine what you want your foundation to accomplish. With your answers as your guide, you'll be able to choose a foundation that meets your individual needs and is best suited to your skin. Your choice will lay the foundation for your most attractive beauty look.

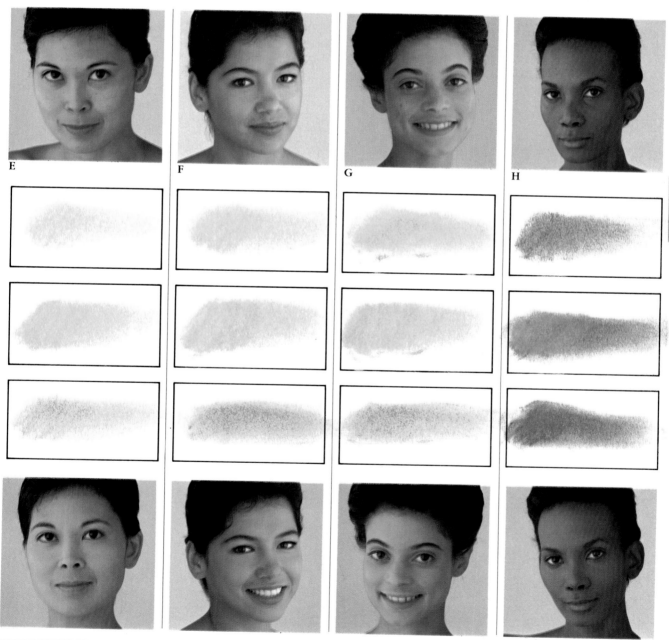

E   F   G   H

Taking a Closer Look

Circle the answers that best describe your skin.

1. The overall coloring of my complexion in bright daylight is:
   A. Light/ivory.
   B. Medium/beige.
   C. Dark/bronze.

2. The underlying tone of the skin on my neck in bright daylight shows subtle hints of:
   A. Pink/blue.
   B. Gold/yellow.

3. Overall, my skin tone is:
   A. Consistent, generally even in color and texture.
   B. Darker around the eyes, nostrils, and mouth.
   C. Uneven — some blotchiness, discoloration, and/or freckling.

4. My skin type is:
   A. Dry.
   B. Normal.
   C. Oily.
   D. Combination.

5. I want my foundation to:
   A. Blend with my skin tone, for the most natural look possible.
   B. Enhance my natural skin tone and coloring, making it appear more golden or more rosy.
   C. Conceal or camouflage, veiling imperfections.

Your answers to statements 1 and 2 are your guide to finding a complementary foundation shade; however, keep in mind that more than one shade will most likely suit your skin tone. The most efficient way to select a makeup base is to try a number of colors before you make a decision.

Your answer to statement 3 indicates the amount of coverage you need from a foundation. If you answered A, your options are open. Base your choice of foundation shade on the look you want to achieve. If, for example, you want a natural or sporty look, choose a foundation that closely matches your skin tone. For a bronze look, select a slightly darker shade; for elegant evenings, you may prefer a slightly lighter base. Because your skin tone is consistent, you can make your selection according to your personal preference.

If your answer was B, you have the same options outlined above. However, before applying your foundation, you will want extra help in concealing darker areas. The corrective techniques explained at right show you how to use yellow foundation to even out your skin tone.

If you answered C, you will also want to follow the corrective procedures at right to camouflage imperfections. After you've completed these steps, you'll achieve a flattering look by selecting an intermediate shade of foundation that blends the various tones in your complexion.

Your skin type, indicated in statement 4, also affects the kind of foundation that will be most beneficial. For optimum coverage and wearability, see pages 50 to 53.

Statement 5 relates to what you want your foundation to achieve. If you answered A, you can attain a natural look by selecting a foundation shade that closely matches and blends well with your skin tone.

Your natural coloring is an important consideration if you answered B. For a sun-warmed effect, choose a more golden shade. And for a look that's more radiant and alive, opt for a foundation with more rose in it.

If your answer is C, you'll want to master the art of corrective makeup to veil imperfections effectively. As a general rule, you can achieve the smoothest look by selecting an intermediate foundation shade.

Remember: you can accomplish the best results by experimenting with a variety of makeup shades. To ensure that you select a flattering shade, always try foundation before you buy.

Highlighting and Concealing

Bringing out a special area of your face is called highlighting, and the way to get the most naturally dramatic results is to use a white foundation under your tinted foundation. You may want to accentuate the pretty shape of your eyes or the lovely high curve of your cheekbones.

Apply white highlighting foundation after daytime moisturizer (if you use a moisturizer) or after you have freshened your skin in the morning, leaving it clean and ready for makeup.

When highlighting your eyes, concentrate on your browbone — the spot right under the outer half of each eyebrow. Dot a very small amount onto the tip of your ring finger, and gently pat it onto the skin in tiny dots. Continue patting until the color is blended, working it out toward the end of your eyebrow. A small dot applied and blended just above the outer corner of your eye will further accentuate your eyes.

You can highlight your cheekbones in much the same way. Find the very top of your cheeks with your fingertips by feeling below the outer corners of your eyes. Apply a very small amount of highlighter to your ring finger and place tiny dots in this area. Continue patting the area to blend in the white foundation, working up toward your temple.

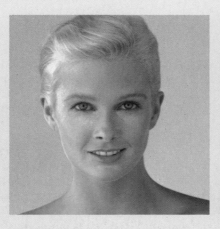
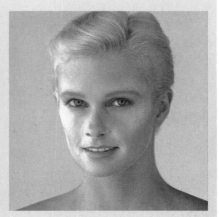

Skin Care

Highlighting works best when it's subtle. Too much white foundation can detract from, rather than enhance, your best features. Even before you apply your skin-toned foundation, highlighting should be so well blended that it is barely discernible. For optimum blendability and protection, the formula of white foundation you use should be the same as the formula of your tinted foundation; use a creamy oil-based foundation for dry and normal skin, an oil-absorbent liquid foundation for combination and oily skin.

In taking the inventory on these pages, you may also have discovered that you would like to blend color irregularities, conceal fine lines or imperfections, or cover up dark or red areas. A yellow foundation, applied before your tinted foundation, works best to conceal flaws and blend coloring irregularities. It is especially useful for eliminating dark areas under the eyes. This concealing foundation should be in the same formula (oil- or water-based) as your tinted foundation to ensure that the two foundations blend.

To conceal minor flaws, take a tiny dot of yellow foundation on your fingertip and pat it right on the spot or area you want to blend and conceal. Still using light patting movements of the fingertip, work outward from the spot or blemish so that the yellow color becomes progressively paler. You should never be able to see a line between the areas where you use yellow foundation and the surrounding skin.

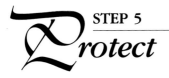

Protect

Protect, the final step in your daily morning skin-care routine, gives your skin a smooth sheen while shielding it from the environment.

Dry and normal skin require a creamy oil-based foundation. Be sure your face is clean. Then to apply your foundation, first moisten your face and neck slightly with either tepid water or moisturizer. (If you prefer to use a daytime moisturizer under your foundation, do not use water. If you moisten your face with water, use your fingertips and dry your hands before applying your cream foundation.) Using a tiny spatula, transfer a small amount of foundation to your fingertips and apply it to one area of your face at a time, following the proper movement of application shown at right. (It's always best to start with as little foundation as possible, since it's easier to apply more where you need it than to remove any excess.) Without pressing or tugging your skin, gently blend in the foundation, using upward and outward strokes. Be sure to spread it up to the hairline and beyond the jawline to prevent lines from showing where the makeup ends. The color should become progressively lighter as you spread the foundation up and out toward your hairline and onto your jaw and neck.

Combination and oily skin need a water-based liquid foundation. Shake the foundation well, then dab it onto your fingertips and apply, blending upward and outward toward your hairline, and onto your jawline and neck until you can't see where your foundation ends. Be sure to use the proper movement of application, as illustrated at the right. For more coverage, apply several thin coats, allowing each one to dry before applying the next one.

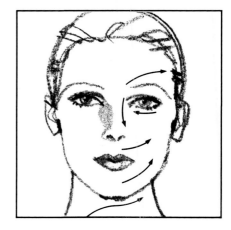

Proper movement of application

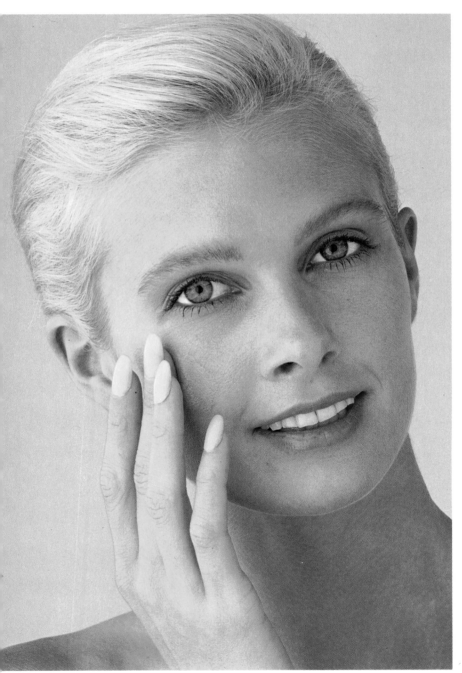

Foundation makes your skin look lovely — even in tone and smooth in texture as it protects. Apply a small amount of foundation to one area of your face at a time. With upward and outward strokes, blend it in gently. Be sure to blend especially well beyond the jawline and all the way to your hairline for a natural look that doesn't show where your foundation ends. Now you're ready to apply the rest of your makeup.

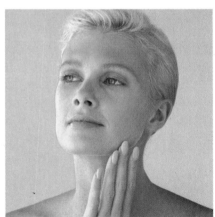

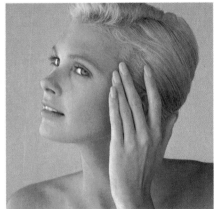

$\mathcal{M}$aking It Yours

If you want to feel beautiful, investing time and effort to care for your skin pays off. You'll find you can have soft and smooth skin that radiates good health: skin that *shows* how well you care for it. All you have to do is establish your own beauty routine and devote a small amount of your time to it every day.

More than any other single factor of beauty care, *consistency* will bring you glowing results. Your skin relies on what *you* do for it to help it function well and look its best. If you're erratic about taking care of it, your skin may respond erratically — possibly with breakouts or extreme oiliness or dryness. That's why it's so important to include the five steps to beautiful skin in your daily schedule — and to perform each step in the proper order:

Step 1: Cleanse The essential first step that removes daily impurities from your facial surface.

Step 2: Stimulate The twice-a-week step that helps improve blood circulation and supplies more oxygen and other nutrients to your skin. This step also removes excess oil that's accumulated and further helps to make your pores appear smaller.

Step 3: Freshen The very important step that removes all traces of cleanser or mask, restores your skin's natural acid balance, and refreshes your whole facial surface.

Step 4: Moisturize The vital step that helps your skin keep its natural water content within the tissues and prevents the loss of precious moisture (one of the most significant elements in keeping your skin young looking).

Step 5: Protect The final step that brings together what's unique about our approach to skin care. Protecting your skin from environmental hazards with foundation gives it the healthful support it needs to face the day, *and* makes it look radiant and even-toned.

You can see from the chart at right how easy and convenient it is to include the five steps to beautiful skin in your daily routine. Good skin care is the essential groundwork for achieving and maintaining the best possible skin, and the basis from which to move on to exciting makeup techniques. So begin your own skin-care routine and make it work for you.

Five easy steps: cleanse, stimulate, freshen, moisturize, and protect. Put them to work for you to achieve the most radiant skin possible. Never miss a day. Never skip a step. Following the right beauty regimen, with the right beauty products, is the best way to keep your skin in optimum condition.

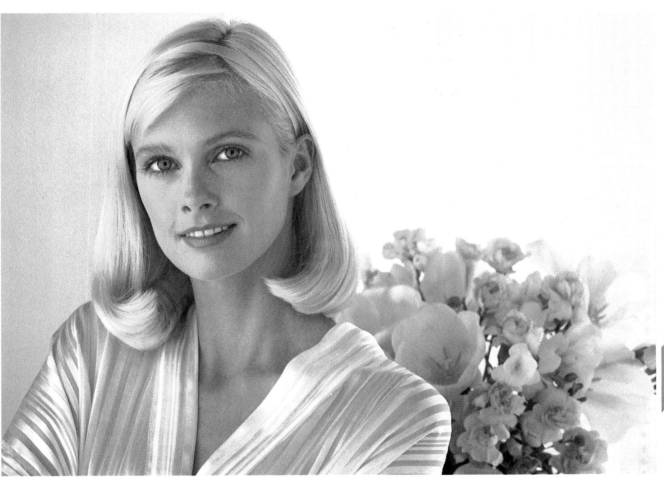

	Dry	Normal	Combination	Oily
STEP 1 Cleanse	Every evening before bed			Morning and evening if desired
STEP 2 Stimulate	Twice a week after cleansing			Twice a week, or more when skin is oilier, after cleansing
STEP 3 Freshen	Every evening after cleansing			
	Twice a week in the evening after masking			In the evening after masking
	Every morning before applying foundation			
STEP 4 Moisturize	Every evening after freshening, with night cream Every morning after freshening, with daytime moisturizer, as needed		In the morning with daytime moisturizer, on drier areas of your face	In the evening and possibly in the morning, on drier areas of your face
STEP 5 Protect	Every morning after moisturizing		Every morning after moisturizing	Every morning after freshening

THREE · Glamour

Your personal style of beauty evolves naturally from effective, ongoing skin care, the basis for the excitement and glamour of makeup. The blush of glowing cheeks, the jewellike hues that add sparkle to your eyes and define and emphasize your every glance. The soft pinks, reds, or corals that add enchantment to your smile. Your makeup can be creative and expressive, a statement of your femininity, or a sultry, sizzling suggestion of your adventuresome self.

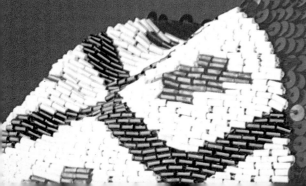

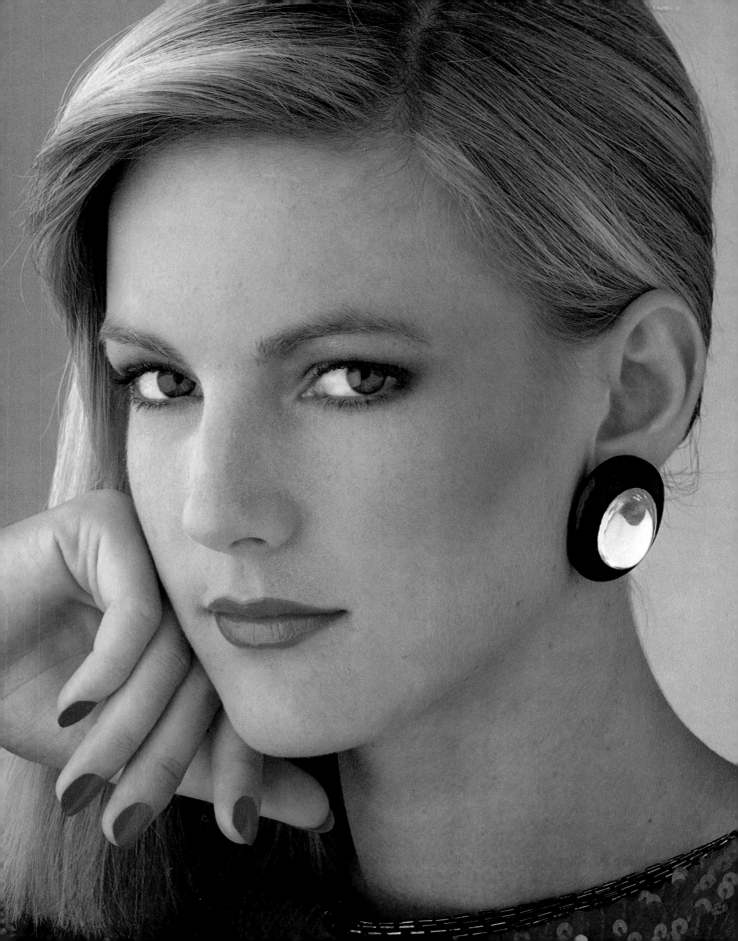

The Magic of Makeup

There's a certain mystique — an unmistakable magic — about makeup. It gives you an instant lift, a confident glow, and a vibrant energy. Cosmetics help you feel polished and put together; they let you define, highlight, and enhance your best features. Even more important, makeup lets you create a full-fashion look that's personalized and up to date, a look that reflects your style, your mood, and your way of life.

Today there are makeup colors, formulas, and application techniques to suit every need and occasion. Never before have so many appealing options been available. Almost magically, a woman looks — and feels — more attractive, more positive, more self-assured.

Makeup also has a positive effect on your psychological well-being. Psychologists have found that makeup can actually enhance a woman's self-esteem and sense of her self-worth. In two different research projects at large universities, psychologists uncovered some startling conclusions about women and cosmetics:

- Women who use makeup have greater self-confidence than those who don't.
- Women who use makeup tend to experience less social anxiety than those who don't.
- Women who do not use makeup tend to avoid social interaction.
- Women who want to affect others positively use makeup and tend to experiment with their cosmetics more often than those who don't.
- Women who use makeup regularly are more satisfied with the appearance of their faces than those who don't.
- Women who wear makeup are more outgoing and more sociable than those who don't.
- Women who wear makeup regularly can anticipate earning as much as 12 percent more than those who don't!

Makeup not only influences the way the world sees you, it has a strong and positive effect on the way you see yourself. Think about your own experience. It's difficult to deny that wearing makeup makes most of us feel better about the way we look and the ways others perceive us. Makeup gives you a finished, well-groomed look that can be as important to your business image as it is to your social life. When you take the time to apply makeup carefully and properly, you tell the world that you like the way you look and that

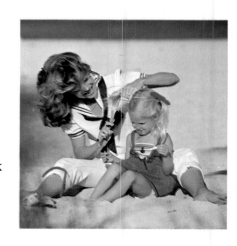

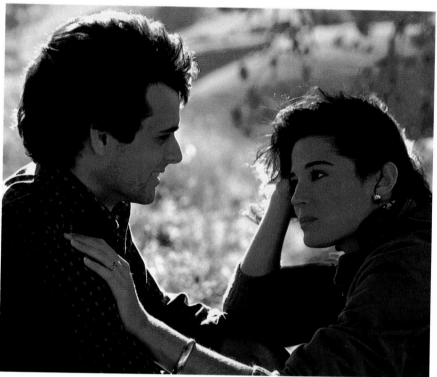

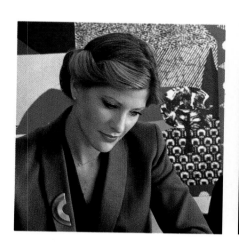

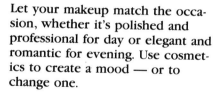

Let your makeup match the occasion, whether it's polished and professional for day or elegant and romantic for evening. Use cosmetics to create a mood — or to change one.

you want to be noticed; it reflects your interest in yourself and your appearance. Confidence generated by your own polished look is a big plus in many situations — it helps you create a good first impression when you apply for a job, meet new people at a party, make a sales presentation that really counts, meet your child's teacher, or go after an important contract or promotion.

Our widely varied daily activities call for a variety of makeup looks. Think of your cosmetics as clothing: a wardrobe of makeup looks to match your different beauty needs. In the following section we provide both the instruction and the inspiration to help you achieve your unique glamour look. We begin with basic daytime glamour makeup. This simple, convenient approach to makeup application and color is flexible enough to suit your daily needs and give you that polished look you want to face your world every day. Special tips for women on the go tell you how to make the transition from a soft, natural daytime look to a dramatic, sophisticated evening look.

Remember: you don't have to be born a perfect beauty to look pretty every day. The key is to experiment, be creative, and have fun with makeup and color. You'll discover that the change in your looks can change your life.

$\mathcal{G}$lamour Basics

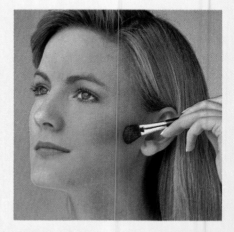

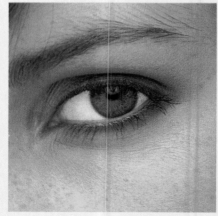

Makeup can make the difference, and in the following pages we tell you how to find your special look and keep it — beautifully. Here is a complete and simple procedure for applying makeup to guide you in creating your own personal look for basic daytime glamour. The tips and techniques are organized in the order we feel makeup is best applied, beginning with cheek and face color for an overall tone. Blusher contours your face with pretty definition, giving it a healthy glow. It also calls attention upward toward your eyes — your most expressive feature. Eye makeup adds a dramatic note and balances the effect of your cheek color. With eyebrow pencil, eye shadow, eyeliner, eye-defining pencil, and mascara you can create a total look that draws others' eyes to yours. You can shape, define, and enhance your eyes for an effect that suits your personal beauty style. Lip color and gloss complete the basic daytime look, adding luster and shine to your mouth. For each of these features we offer basic makeup guidelines plus special tips on how to make the most of various face, eye, and lip shapes. There's even a special section on color to help you learn what shades of blusher, eye makeup, and lip color are best for your coloring.

Once you've learned the glamour basics — the simple steps to your beautiful daytime look — we invite you to experiment and have some fun with an exciting plunge into the world of makeup. Beginning on page 114 we guide you through dozens of exciting and creative makeup looks. All you need are the Glamour Basics and your cosmetics — your ticket to a Glamour Adventure!

Begin your daytime Glamour Basics by adding color to your cheeks, using cream rouge and/or powder blusher. Eye shadow, in glorious shades or subdued neutral hues, contours your eyes and adds a touch of sophistication and everyday elegance.

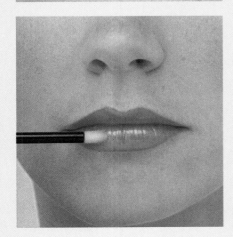

Mascara is the final touch for sparkling eyes; brush it on your top and bottom eyelashes to add color, thickness, and length. Pull your total daytime glamour look together with lip color, first defining the shape of your mouth with a lipliner pencil, then filling in with color and adding a final glimmer of gloss.

Caring for Your Makeup

Almost all cosmetics that contain coloring agents are sensitive to ultraviolet and visible radiation; keep them out of direct sun and away from windows. In addition, dampness can affect both powder-based and cream-based makeup. High humidity causes powders to crumble or it may create the ideal conditions for mold to form on cream-based cosmetics. Cosmetics will last longer and stay fresher if you keep them on a vanity table in your bedroom, rather than in the bathroom where you shower.

Never leave cosmetics in your car in very cold or very hot weather. When you travel by plane, carry your cosmetics with you rather than packing them in your checked luggage. Keep your cosmetics away from drafty windows, heating ducts, or air-conditioning outlets.

Containers should always be closed securely to protect contents from dust or environmental soils, and be sure to wash your hands before using cosmetics. Clean cosmetic brushes after you use them. Lip, blending, eye, blusher, and powder brushes should be carefully wiped clean with a tissue. Eye-shadow brushes should be rinsed with tepid water and gently dried with a tissue when they become soiled. Once a month wash your brushes in mild detergent and rinse them with tepid water. Be sure to dry them thoroughly before storing. A cool, dry storage place for brushes will help them last longest.

All disposable items for makeup application — cotton balls or cotton swabs, for example — should be kept in closed containers to keep them clean. Do not use them more than once.

Taking a Closer Look

Choosing the most flattering makeup colors and making them yours should be based on many factors: the colors of your clothing, the occasion, the season, the time of day, and even your mood. But to make the best color choices in makeup you must understand your natural coloring. The next four pages can help you decide what color range in makeup will be most complimentary to you.

People simplify the way they describe their coloring by looking at the composite tones of their skin and hair — the largest areas of natural coloring. The next most important consideration is eye color, which is also obvious. One way to select makeup shades is to find those that enhance your natural coloring. Another approach is to wear dramatic — and perhaps unexpected — complements.

As a general rule, every woman can wear almost any color. The secret is finding the most flattering variation of a color and the appropriate range of intensity. If you look closely in a well-lighted mirror, you will discover many colors in your hair, skin, and eyes. Skin is not a single flat color; it has a translucent quality and can be affected by discoloration (from blemishes, marks, and veins). As a result, when light is reflected on your face, you may find several hues within a small area. In addition, you'll see many different-colored strands in your hair and flecks of more than one color in your eyes, with a darker shade outlining the iris.

You can bring out those colors through the creative use of makeup — highlighting your natural coloring. Today, there are no rules concerning cosmetic shades. Wear the colors that make you look and feel wonderfully radiant. On pages 86 and 87 the eight women pictured are wearing makeup shades selected for them by scientific measurement — colors well suited to their individual coloring. As you'll see, however, we have included a range of shades from each color group that each woman can wear successfully. These colors work because they're the right intensity: they're compatible with each person's natural coloring.

Color should be fun. It should add interest and excitement to your makeup. Use color to express your moods; see how different colors make you feel when you wear them, how they affect your spirit, your attitude, your enthusiasm. Be adventurous, daring, and inventive. Try as many different combinations as you can. Then choose your favorites to help you make your personal makeup statement.

Use this color spectrum to help guide you in selecting the most flattering intensities of colors for you. Try blending and highlighting (special highlighter shades are ideal for this purpose) and mixing and matching to give mood and magic to your look.

Color your world — and discover that the options are unlimited. That's because there are so many sensational shades of eye, lip, and cheek colors to choose from. Blue isn't just blue. It's also midnight, sky, royal, and more. Green might be kelly, mint, or emerald; red becomes brick, ruby, or rose.

Most important, remember that you can wear any color that strikes your fancy — the key is selecting the color intensities that are right for you. The chart below can help you identify those shades. Keep in mind that the examples here are just a sampling of the wide spectrum available to you — a few of the many hues well suited to your coloring. To find those shades, identify the model on the following two pages whose skin tone most closely resembles your own. (Again, these are just a limited number of the colorations possible.) If your coloring resembles model A, B, C, or D, you can successfully wear any of the colors marked 1 through 8 on the chart. If you resemble model E, F, G, or H, your best colors are marked 9 through 14.

Now, select your favorites. Once you get started, you'll discover that a few basic shades can blossom into a beautiful garden of color!

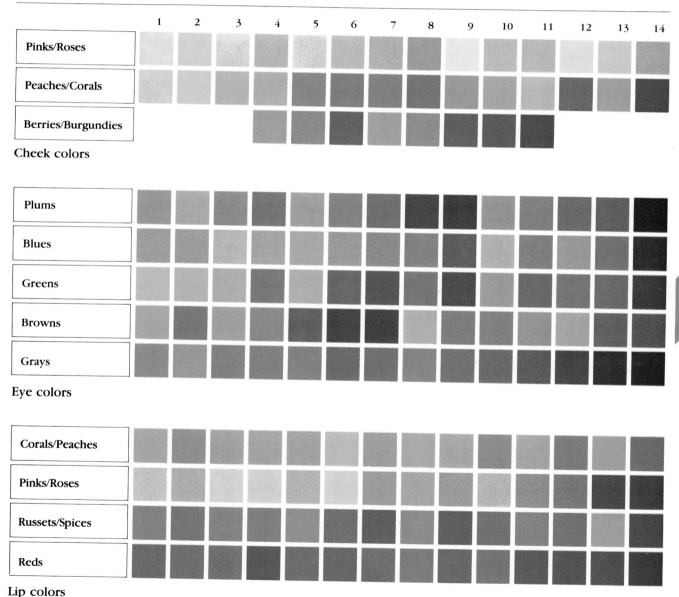

Cheek colors

Eye colors

Lip colors

Glamour

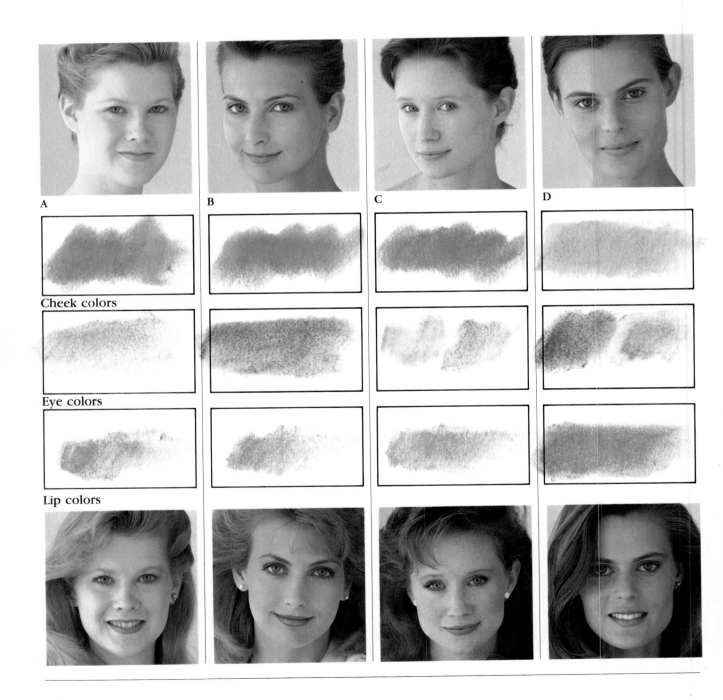

A

B

C

D

Cheek colors

Eye colors

Lip colors

E   F   G   H

Blusher

The color and intensity of your makeup scheme is based on your cheek color, so applying it, in two steps, is the logical beginning of a basic daytime makeup look. First, use a cream rouge to brighten and define the shape of your face and give prominence to your eyes and the contours of your face. Then use a powder blusher on top to give your face a matte finish. Powder blusher over cream rouge also deepens your cheek coloring and helps it last longer. Cream rouge by itself gives a fresh, dewy surface to dry skin, although if you have oily skin you shouldn't use cream rouge at all.

Although cream rouges come in many shades, red cream rouge serves most women best as a basic color. Your powder blusher then enhances and deepens your cheek color. If you don't use a red cream rouge, use a powder blusher in the same tone range as your cream rouge.

If you use only powder blusher you can be somewhat more adventurous in choosing a color. Powder blusher allows your skin's natural color to blend with your cheek color. You will find, however, that the same color blusher looks and blends differently on different skin tones. As a result, the best way to achieve the look you want is to experiment with many shades to see which ones give you the desired results — a natural blush, a bright tone, or a soft, warm color.

Two similar shades of blusher are often packaged together. Use the lighter shade to give the top of your cheekbone a glowing blush color, and the darker one to contour the area under your cheekbone. (See the directions on how to apply powder blusher on pages 90 and 91.) When selecting two shades to be used together, be sure they are within the same color range — pinks, peaches, or berries — to allow for proper blending.

To achieve a *natural blush,* stay within the realm of your natural skin tones; refer to your color inventory on page 84 for help in choosing compatible cheek color. If your natural coloring is in the pink/blue range, you should select a pink or rose for your cheeks; if your coloring is gold/yellow, select a soft coral or peach tone to give your cheeks a natural blush look.

To *brighten* your skin tone, use a blusher slightly darker than the natural color of your skin. For example, if your skin is pale, you need a cheek color in delicate rose or berry tones. Medium-depth

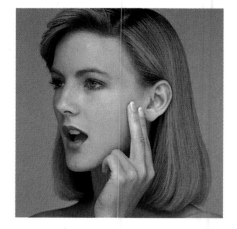

To find the hollow of your cheek, place your finger on your cheekbone where it intersects with your jawbone. Now open your mouth; you should be able to feel where the two bones are hinged. Slip your fingertip down into the area just below that intersection — that's the hollow of your cheek.

skin tones can be brightened with clear reds and strong berry shades. The darker your skin, the more intense your cheek color should be — perhaps deep berry shades with hints of burgundy.

To *warm and soften* your skin tone, your cheek color should contain soft golden shades. If you have pale skin, find a gentle peach shade for cheeks; medium-toned skin blends with deep peach to coral hues; and dark skin needs the deep golden corals to add the warm softness you want.

What is most important when choosing cheek color is matching the *intensity* of your natural coloring — not too pale, not too dark. Of course, the best method for choosing a color is experimentation — try various shades to find the colors that work best for you.

Applying Cream Rouge

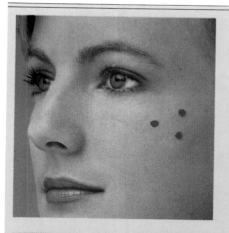

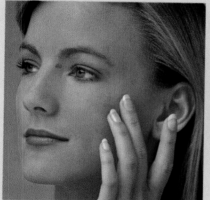

As a base for powder blusher, classic red cream rouge enhances your cheek makeup and allows your overall color to last longer. To apply cream rouge, begin by looking straight into a well-lighted mirror. Find the top ridge of your cheekbone, directly below the pupil of your eye. Place a tiny dot of cream rouge on your fingertip and apply the dot to that area.

Next, feel along the top ridge of your cheekbone to the edge that is under the outer corner of your eye (imagine a straight line drawn from the eye's outer corner to the top of the cheekbone). Apply another small dot of cream rouge to this spot.

Then, feel for the bottom ridge of your cheekbone, which should be at the same level as the bottom of your nose (imagine a straight line drawn from the bottom of your nostril out to your cheek); this spot should be directly below the dot you've just applied under the outer corner of your eye. Apply a third dot there.

Your dots of cream rouge should form a triangle on your cheek as shown here. Wipe the excess rouge from your fingertips and gently blend the dots with an outward movement toward your ears. Shortly after applying your cream rouge, check to see how much color is still apparent. If it looks too bright, wipe the excess rouge off gently. Oily skin tends to make cream cheek color disappear more readily, so if your skin is oily, use powder blusher.

Blusher & Face Powder

Powder blusher gives your face extra depth and a radiant glow to enhance your daytime look. Powder blusher over cream rouge adds a deeper tone to your cheek color and helps it last longer. When used alone, powder blusher allows your natural skin tone to come through while adding a matte finish to your cheeks.

Tips on how to apply powder blusher are covered at right. Depending on your face shape you may want to modify some of these instructions to enhance or downplay your own features (see pages 92 to 95). Whatever your face shape, though, proper blending is most important in applying blusher. There should be no line of separation between the lighter and darker shades. In blending even a single color of blusher, the intensity of color should lessen gradually outward toward your ears, so it doesn't end abruptly at your hairline or upper jaw. Using a blending or blusher brush for blending can be helpful in achieving the soft, natural look you want from powder blusher. Stroke the blending brush repeatedly over the area where the two shades of blusher combine, brushing in an upward and outward movement until your cheek color blends perfectly with surrounding skin tones.

Translucent Face Powder Applied after cream cheek color, and before or after powder blusher, translucent face powder adds a smooth matte finish to your skin and helps blend your cheek color with your natural skin tone. Translucent powder does not significantly add to or alter the color of your foundation; it merely evens out the texture of your skin. Thus, the shade of powder you choose should complement your natural coloring and foundation shade.

Apply face powder with either a brush or a puff. Gently stroke the brush or puff across the cake of powder, then apply it lightly over your face and neck, using downward movements (in the same direction facial hair grows) to distribute the powder evenly. A small amount applied very lightly to your eyes (close each eye and brush gently over the lid) helps blend the texture in this area with that of the surrounding skin. It also helps eye makeup last longer. Face powder gives a final polish to your skin, smoothing its surface and "setting" foundation and cheek color.

For oily skin, translucent powder helps absorb surface oil, reduce shine, and keep makeup looking fresh.

To apply powder blusher, stroke the brush tip evenly across the cake of blusher, shake or tap off any excess blusher, and begin applying color at the hollow of your cheek (see page 88). Then use the brush to gently blend the color out toward your ears. Or brush powder blusher smoothly across your cheeks, either by itself or over cream rouge. A good general rule is that blusher should never be closer to your nose than the width of two fingers.

To apply two colors of blusher, stroke the brush tip lightly across the lighter-colored powder and brush it on the top of your cheekbone, where you want the most intense color. Begin just under the outer corner of each eye and brush inward with light, blending strokes to gradually lighten the density of color toward your lower cheek, level with the bottom of your nose. To apply the darker shade of blusher, first wipe your brush clean with a tissue, then stroke it evenly over the darker-colored cake. Begin applying your blusher in the hollow of your cheek, blending upward and outward into the lighter shade you've already applied.

To apply translucent face powder, use a brush or a puff to cover your face. Be sure to use gentle downward strokes.

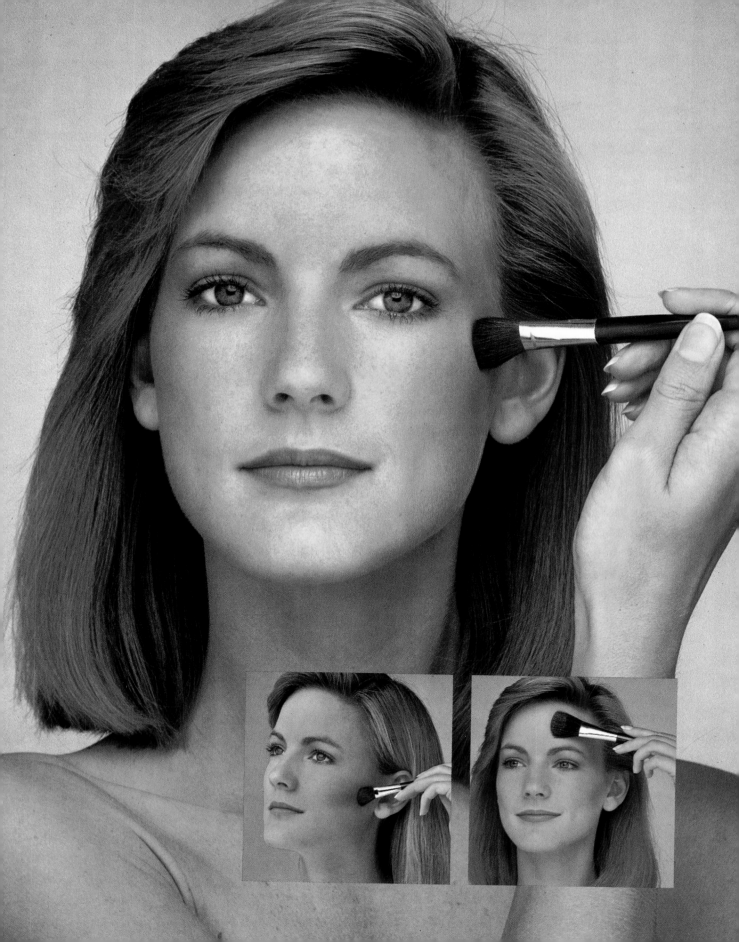

Taking a Closer Look

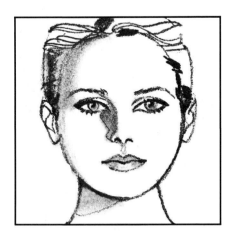 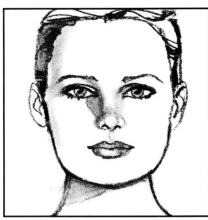 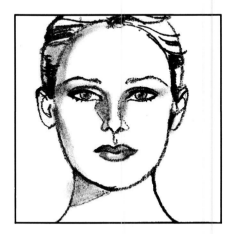

If the shape of your face is **round**, you can elongate it by using a single shade of blusher in V-shapes, forming crescents around your outer eye area. Begin by sweeping the blusher lightly onto your cheekbones, at a level just above your nostrils, at the midpoint of your cheeks. Bring the color up around your temple, from outside the outer corner of your eye, and extend it onto your forehead, just above the arch of each eyebrow. Last, stroke a small amount of blusher on the midpoint of your chin.

If your jaw and brow are wide and your face has a **rectangular** or squared-off appearance, you can round and soften these contours with blusher. Start the blusher at the middle of each cheek, on a level just above your nostrils, below the outer edge of your iris. Sweep color up and out on your temples, tapering off on a level even with the tops of your eyelids. Blend blusher well into the area where your hairline begins. Then softly brush a small wisp of blusher on the point of your chin and high in the center of your forehead.

If your face is an elongated **oval** and you think it appears too long, you can shorten its appearance. Begin by applying cream rouge in the three-dot triangle method demonstrated on page 89. Then use powder blusher to intensify the cream rouge color. Also add light strokes of blusher over the bridge of your nose, along the middle of your brow, and across your chin. This sun-kissed look adds horizontal contours to your face and shortens its appearance.

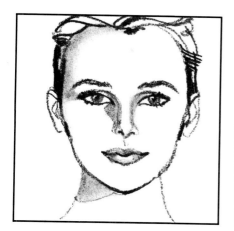

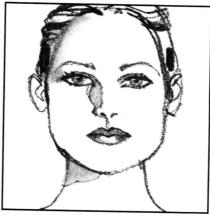

If you have a narrow jaw and wide cheeks, giving your face a triangular or **heart-shaped** look, you can use highlighter (white foundation in a formula compatible with your skin type; see page 73) and powder blusher to balance the width of the upper and lower parts of your face. Begin by dotting a small amount of highlighter at the corners of your jaw and in the center of your chin; blend well into your foundation. Next, apply blusher in a crescent shape, beginning just above the arch of each eyebrow and bringing the color down over your temple area at the outer corners of your eyes and on your cheekbones at a level just above your nostrils. Continue the color into the center of each cheek, just below the pupil of the eye. This will make your cheek area appear slimmer and your jaw wider.

If a broad jaw and narrow forehead give your face a **diamond-shaped** contour, you can compensate for this shape by using highlighter, powder blusher, and contour blusher. Begin by dotting a small amount of highlighter above each eyebrow, midway between your brows and hairline; blend the highlighter well into your foundation. Next, apply blusher, beginning at the very top of your cheekbones, sweeping the color out toward your ears so it extends from the area outside the outer corners of your eyes down below your earlobes. Then dot a small amount of blusher on the point of your chin. Next, begin blending the contour shade of blusher into your cheek color at earlobe level, and extend the contour down to the square point of your jaw. Be sure to blend well to avoid an obvious line along your jawline.

Choosing Glasses

Eyeglasses are an important fashion accessory today. When you select eyeglass frames, be sure they are proportionate in size to your face; the upper perimeters should not extend above your eyebrows. The right frames can actually enhance the contours of your face. The secret lies in knowing how various sizes and shapes of eyeglass frames affect the way you look. Oval or circular frames help round the curves of an angular face, softening a square jaw or protruding cheekbones. Square frames add needed angles to a round or full face, giving definition to ample contours. Aviator frames — asymmetrical ovals with the broadest part resting toward the outer areas of the face below the corners of the eyes — add fullness to the lower face and give symmetry to a narrow or pointed chin. Upswept oval frames that are widest at the temples, above the outer corners of the eyes, can make the eyes appear farther apart and the brow area broader. Such frames are flattering to a narrow face or one with a proportionally wide jaw. Wide-bridged frames create the impression of a slimmer face, especially if the outer edges of the frames extend beyond the temples. Low-bridged frames tend to shorten or minimize a long or large nose.

If you wear glasses, you'll want to take advantage of the extra attention they focus on your eyes by using the very best eye makeup techniques. Draw attention toward the lower areas of your eyes, to balance the upper eyes and brows accentuated by most eyeglass frames.

Glamour

Taking a Closer Look

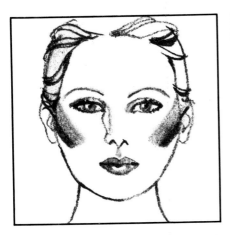
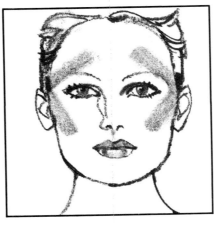
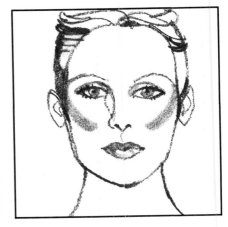

If your cheeks seem too **rounded** — not prominent or angular enough — try using powder blusher, contour blusher, and highlighter (white foundation in a formula compatible with your skin type; see page 73). Begin by feeling for the very top of each cheekbone. Apply a small amount of highlighter there, blending it into your foundation. Just below the highlighter, sweep on your powder blusher, stroking the color from your upper cheek inward and downward to a level even with your nostrils. Next, stroke on the contour shade of your powder blusher either below or on the outer side of your blusher, so that the color begins just above your earlobe and is applied in a downward and inward movement to a level even with your nostrils. Then, using a clean blending brush, blend the blusher and contour shade with an upward and outward stroke so the different shades of the cheek color blend well with each other and with your skin.

If you think your cheeks are too **full and widely spaced,** you will probably want to make your upper face appear slimmer and your cheeks less broad. To achieve both these effects, apply a single shade of cream rouge or blusher cheek color in a V-shape, beginning high on each upper cheekbone near the outer corner of your eye, where you will want the greatest intensity of color. Bring the point of the V down to the level of your cheek parallel with your nostrils, under the pupil of your eye. Extend the opposite angle of the V upward toward the inner corner of each eye, stopping at a level parallel with the middle of your nose.

If your cheeks seem too **close together** and your upper face looks too narrow, you can add fullness by using a single cheek color. First apply highlighter just outside the outer corner of each eye, above your cheekbone. After blending foundation highlighter into your foundation, apply cheek color — either cream rouge or blusher — beginning at the temple area outside the outer corner of each eye, bringing the color down over your outer cheek. Taper it off in a slightly rounded U-shape toward your nose, on a level with your nostrils.

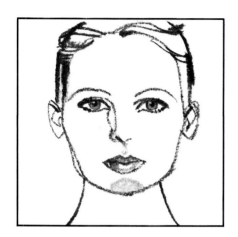

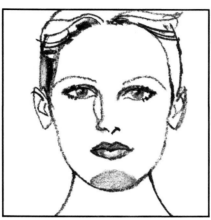

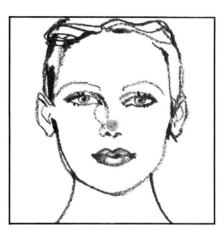

Makeup techniques can also help you change the appearance of your nose and chin. If your ***chin recedes*** too much, apply tiny dots of highlighter, forming a crescent over your chin. Blend the highlighter lightly downward and inward toward the center of your chin to make it appear more prominent.

If your ***chin protrudes*** too much, you can make it seem smaller and less prominent by applying a contour shade of blusher in a crescent over the bottom of your chin. Blend the contour shade well so it doesn't form an obvious line (extend the color down under your chin), and make sure it doesn't have a muddy appearance.

Contouring or highlighting to change the shape of your ***nose*** is difficult even for professional makeup artists. However, try dotting highlighter very lightly on the tip of your nose to lengthen a short nose, or applying a small amount of darker foundation on the tip of your nose to make a long nose appear less prominent. The most effective way to improve the shape or size of your nose is to de-emphasize it. Draw attention elsewhere: to your eyes by eye shadowing and eye defining; or to your cheeks by applying cheek color above your eyebrows, on your temples, and outside your cheekbones. Give prominence to your cheekbones by using contour blusher shades. Try pale, subtle shades of lip color, and sweep a small amount of powder blusher over your chin.

Eyebrow Pencil

Eyebrows frame your eyes and add expression to your entire face. On most women one eyebrow has a "better" shape than the other — a more natural arc or a smoother line. Decide which of your eyebrows is better and use it as a guide for shaping the other one. The natural shape you want can be achieved by tweezing, waxing (see below), or using an eyebrow pencil.

An eyebrow pencil is used to add shape and fullness to eyebrows. It should have a fine point for easy application and soft lead for a soft, natural line. Eyebrow pencils come in a wide variety of shades, so you can select one to match your natural eyebrow coloring or hair coloring perfectly. The color should never be darker than that of your brows or hair color, unless you have very light-colored hair.

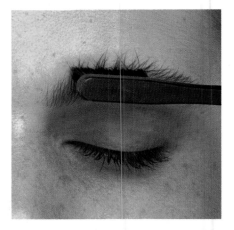

Shaping Your Eyebrows

Tweezing is an excellent way to thin brows that are too bushy. *Never* pull out hairs above the natural line of your eyebrows; tweeze only brow hairs under your eyebrows, on the bridge of your nose, or beyond the outer corners of your eyes. (Take care not to thin your eyebrows too much; the delicate hair follicles in this area can be destroyed by tweezing, and hair may not grow back.)

When you tweeze, follow the guidelines for determining eyebrow shape, as illustrated at far right. Wash your tweezers with mild detergent and rinse them well. Then dampen a facecloth with very warm water and hold it gently against the area to be tweezed; this cleans the area and opens the follicles slightly so that tweezing is easier and less painful. Look into a well-lighted mirror and tweeze out the unwanted brow hairs one at a time, rinsing the tweezers periodically to remove clinging hairs.

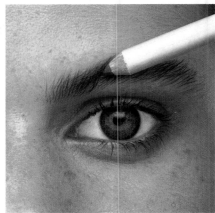

Another option for shaping brows is *waxing* the stray hairs that grow below the eyebrow. Don't try to do it yourself because it can be dangerous to use hot wax so near your eyes; many beauty salons offer the service at reasonable prices.

Eyebrow waxing is done by applying small amounts of liquid molten wax with a narrow brush to the area right under the brows. When the wax dries and hardens, it is peeled off, removing stray hairs by pulling them out of their follicles. The area will be red for a few hours after waxing, so it is best to wait until the following day to apply eye shadow. Because full regrowth after waxing takes about six to eight weeks, you may want to tweeze some stray brow hairs between treatments.

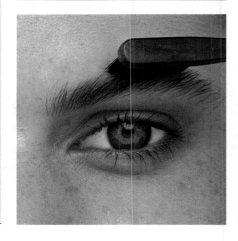

To apply eyebrow pencil, begin by brushing your eyebrows with an eyebrow brush, using quick, upward strokes to remove excess foundation or face powder. Brushing the hairs up also allows you to see their natural color and shape clearly. Then, with outward brush strokes, smooth the hairs in the direction in which they grow.

Now, hold your eyebrow pencil upright so it intersects the inner corner of your eye in a straight line (see photo at right and 1 in diagram below); this is where your eyebrow should begin. If yours falls short of this line, use light, short, feathering strokes of the pencil to fill in your brow.

Next, hold the pencil at an angle so it touches the outer edge of your nostril and intersects with the outer corner of your eye (2); this is where your eyebrow should end. Then hold the pencil parallel to your eye across the bridge of your nose so the inner and outer ends of your brow intersect (3). Your eyebrow should end at the same level at which it begins, or it may be slightly higher than the beginning of your brow. Your eyebrow's outer end should never droop below the inner one.

Now, hold your pencil upright, intersecting the outer edge of the iris of your eye and the middle of your eyebrow (4). This is the point at which the brow should arch highest. The end of your eyebrow, above the outer corner of your eye, should never be higher than this arch, and the ends of both brows should be on an even level.

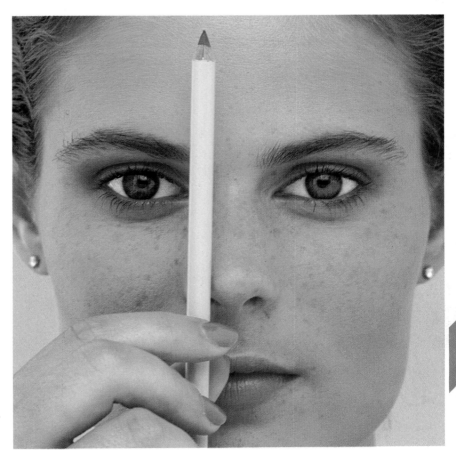

To shape your brows properly, begin by using short, light strokes of the pencil to outline the top of each eyebrow up to its arch. Use featherlike strokes to extend each brow to the end. Fill in any sparse areas by using these same strokes, as though drawing on individual brow hairs. Then brush your brows with an eyebrow brush to smooth them and blend in the pencil strokes.

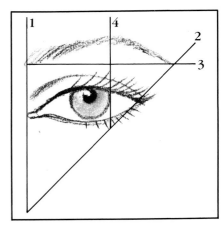

Eye Shadow

Eye shadow is instant magic. Because your eyes are your most expressive facial feature, enhancing them with color and contour can change your face dramatically. For a daytime look, eye shadow should be subtle — it should whisper, not shout, the message your eyes convey.

To achieve the perfect daytime look with eye shadow, you need follow only a few basic guidelines. When you are going to be in bright, natural daylight most of the time, take care to control the *intensity* of your eye shadow color. The shades you choose can be deep-toned or pale, neutral or bright, but they should be applied so that they are not too strong. Blending is the key to achieving the soft glow of color you want from eye shadow. When you use more than one shade they should be so well blended that you can't tell where one ends and the next one begins.

Daytime eyes should be contoured naturally. Look carefully at your eyes to note which areas are naturally highlighted and which are naturally shaded. Then apply light colors to the highlighted areas, such as the browbone, and darker colors to the shaded areas, such as the eyelid crease.

Follow your personal preference in choosing daytime eye shadow colors, but make sure they do not clash with your facial makeup or your clothing. Try to keep all shades in the same family: if you wear soft corals, peaches, orange, and yellow, they are best enhanced with eye colors in the brown range. Bright pink and blue-toned shades (including plum tones) are best set off by eye colors in the blue family.

Using eye shadow that brings out your eyes' natural coloring is an excellent way to create a soft daytime look. You don't have to match your eye tone exactly, but the shade you apply closest to your eye itself — on your eyelid — can pick up one of the secondary tones in your eyes for a beautiful, sparkling, natural effect; green eyes may have golden yellow flecks, brown eyes often have hazel tones, and blue eyes may have highlights of turquoise or violet.

Eye shadow instantly transforms your eyes into vibrant bouquets of color. And learning to apply eye shadow artfully is easy — with a little practice you'll soon be able to achieve a complete wardrobe of eye looks.

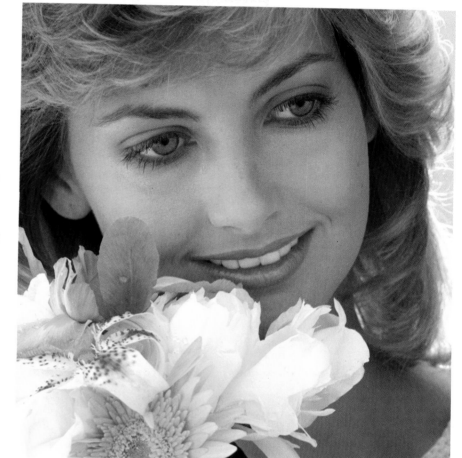

To help you follow the directions for eye makeup application, this diagram names the various parts of the eye area.

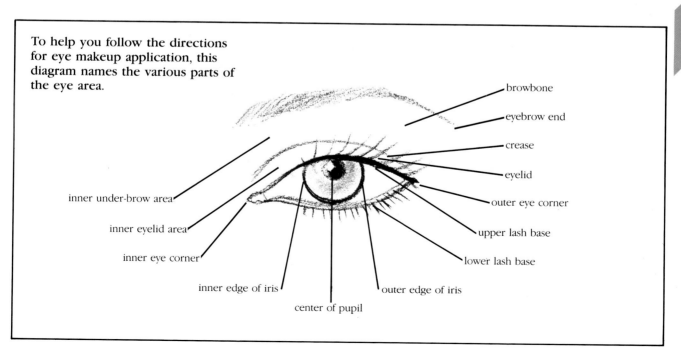

browbone

eyebrow end

crease

eyelid

outer eye corner

upper lash base

lower lash base

inner under-brow area

inner eyelid area

inner eye corner

inner edge of iris

center of pupil

outer edge of iris

Eye Shadow

You may select daytime eye-shadow colors according to the guidelines on pages 98 and 99, but the basic *tones* you need are:

- a pale highlighter shade for your browbone area
- a basic shade for your eyelids

When you apply daytime eye shadow, have the right tools at hand. You'll need:

- a clean, soft, straight-bristled brush, about one-eighth inch wide, for each color you use
- a full, round-bristled brush, about one-half inch wide, for blending eye shadow

Eye shadow comes in three basic types, each with its own special qualities.

Eye shadow in *pressed powder* form that is applied wet with a moistened brush lasts longest and can produce the greatest range in color intensity. Simply moisten a brush with water, then apply the still-moist color to your eyelids, blending quickly before it dries on your skin. You can produce either a sheer translucent color or a richer color by varying the amount of water you mix with the eye shadow. Water-mixed eye shadow stays put for a long time without smudging or forming lines in the creases of your eyes.

Eye shadow in pressed powder form that is applied dry must be used more sparingly, since the color tends to be deeper and more opaque. Apply this eye shadow with a dry eye-shadow brush or sponge-tip applicator, and blend it with a clean blending brush.

Cream eye shadow in cake or stick form is the most intense in color. It may be difficult to use this type of eye shadow if your skin is oily, as the natural oils in your skin may cause it to run. Its texture causes cream eye shadow to look shiny and smudge easily. Apply and blend it with a brush or your fingertip, or use the stick form directly from the tube with its sponge-tip wand applicator.

When you apply eye shadow, always start with the palest shade — the highlighter shadow. Brush it just under the outer end of each eyebrow and quickly blend the color inward toward the inner end of your eyebrow, above the inner corner of your eye. (Blending inward places the most intense color right on your browbone, while the color gradually becomes less intense toward the inner end of your eyebrow.)

Next, apply the eyelid shadow by beginning in the center of each lid, just above the pupil of your eye. With the blending brush, use a quick back-and-forth motion to blend inward toward the inside corner and outward toward the outer corner of each eye. Finish by blending upward to meet the highlighter shade.

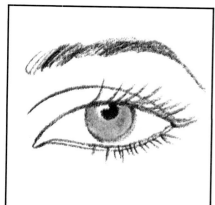

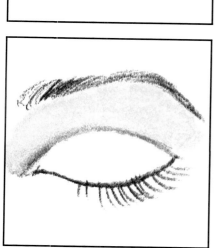

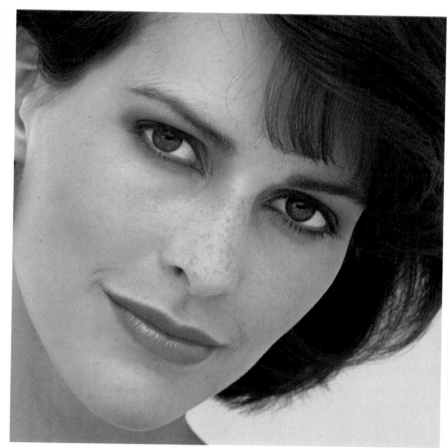

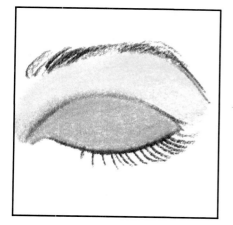

Eye Definers

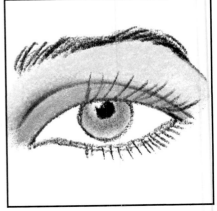

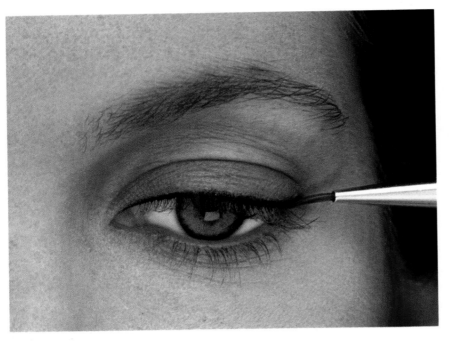

The *eyeliner* you choose should have a quick-drying liquid formula. For easy application, select one in a convenient-to-use tube with a narrow, tapered brush attached to the cap.

To apply eyeliner, draw the brush out of the tube and stroke it against the mouth of the tube to remove excess liquid and taper the brush to a fine point. Then tilt your head back slightly so you are looking down into a mirror and can see your eyelid clearly. Open your mouth slightly to relax your face (this helps to keep eyes still and prevent rapid blinking), and brace your little finger against your cheek to stabilize the brush.

Now, using the very tip of the brush, stroke the eyeliner evenly across your lid as close to the base of your lashes as possible, beginning with the inner corner of your eye and continuing to the outer corner of your eyelid. Apply the line in several short brush strokes.

Whereas eye shadow adds color, contour, and enhancement, lining and defining your eyes accentuate their actual shape. Lining and defining your eyes emphasize their natural setting and contours and make your lashes look thicker. You may use shadow alone for a daytime look, but you can see from the photographs above and at right that lining and defining give a polished, finished look to your daytime eye makeup. Because both lining and defining your eyes take precision and control, you may have to practice these techniques. But you'll find you can quickly master applying both liner and eye-defining pencils for an effect that enhances your finished daytime makeup look. Eyelining is done with black or brown eyeliner on the top lid of each eye, and sometimes under the lower lashes. Blondes, redheads, and light brunettes should use a brown eyeliner, while darker brunettes and those who have black hair should use black eyeliner.

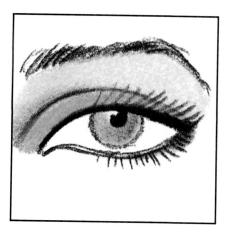

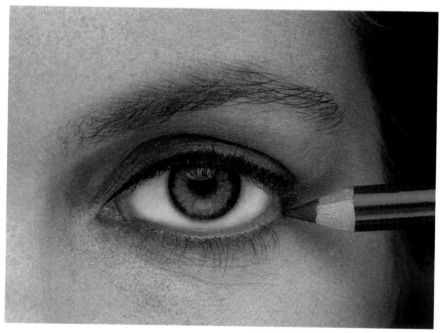

An ***eye-defining pencil***, which is available in a variety of colors, adds definition and a hint of color to the bottom of each eye area. The pencil should have a fine point and a medium to soft lead so it glides on easily under your lower eyelashes. (It's a good idea to have a sharpener you use only for your eye-defining pencil, to keep the point sharp, and to clean the tip before each use.)

To use your eye-defining pencil, lightly stroke a single, fine line under your lower lashes, as close to the base as possible, starting at the outer corner of your eye. Run the pencil smoothly under your lashes along each lower eyelid to the inner corners of your eyes — stopping a short space away from the inner corner. Then use an angled brush or a cotton swab to soften and blend the line. Eye defining should be a light hint of color under your eyes; it should never be a hard, thick line.

Mascara

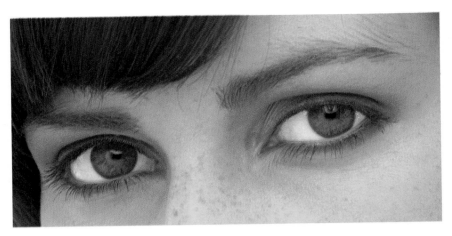

Your eyelashes softly frame your eyes, and adding mascara darkens and thickens your lashes to give your eye makeup the finishing touch. Many women consider mascara to be *the* essential makeup they wear — no matter what the occasion. And it's easy to understand why. Mascara softly accentuates the natural shape and setting of your eyes, bringing out their color and expressiveness.

Mascara packaged in a tube with a fine spiral brush applicator is easy to apply; it curls your eyelashes as it adds color and fullness. Select a neutral shade of mascara — a brown or black — that's compatible with your coloring. Some women make the common mistake of choosing a mascara that's too dark. If your lashes are brown and your eyes are pale, deep black mascara can look harsh and detract from the softness your eyes should convey. Mascara should darken your eyelashes, not change their natural color.

Even smudge-resistant and waterproof mascara may wear off a bit during the day. An occasional extra touch of mascara on the tips of your lashes can do wonders to brighten up your look, so carry your mascara with you wherever you go. For best results, always keep the cap securely closed to keep the mascara from drying out and to prevent contamination, and never share mascara with anyone.

Apply mascara by looking straight into your mirror, with your chin lifted slightly so you can see your lashes clearly. Open your mouth a bit to relax your face. Supporting your elbow on a table or vanity while you apply the mascara helps keep your hand steady.

Gently twist the spiral brush as you withdraw it from the tube case. Never pump your mascara brush up and down in the tube; this distributes the mascara unevenly on the brush and often breaks its bristles. It can also dry out the mascara faster. Stroke your upper lashes evenly from their base to the tips, curling them upward with the brush as you apply the mascara. If your lashes are very light in color you may want to begin applying mascara to the tips, then stroke the lashes from underneath. The initial application to the tips may help you see the lashes better.

Reinsert the brush in the tube and apply mascara to your lower lashes with downward strokes, wiggling the brush back and forth a bit to separate the lashes. After you have applied the mascara to both eyes, you can repeat the application to add more fullness to your eyelashes. If your eyelashes are thick and grow close together, they may clump together when you apply mascara. Allow the mascara to dry, then use the corner of your eyebrow brush to carefully separate your eyelashes.

If your eyelashes are difficult to curl, you may want to consider using an eyelash curler. Use it gently after each application of mascara.

Removing Waterproof Mascara

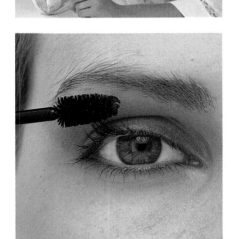

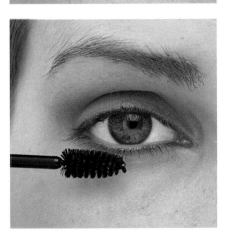

Waterproof mascara is practical for many active women. It has more holding power than the regular formula, which is beneficial if you live in a hot, humid climate or if you like to swim with your makeup on. Because waterproof mascara is not water soluble, it might not come off with your normal cleansing routine. To take it off in the evening before cleansing your face, it is necessary to use a special oil-based, waterproof-mascara remover to dissolve the mascara gently while conditioning your lashes and surrounding skin.

To remove waterproof mascara, apply a small amount of remover to a piece of sterile cotton or a clean cotton ball. Then, very gently, wipe the cotton over each closed eye, stroking downward and outward. Continue to apply the remover until the cotton shows no traces of mascara. Always stroke very lightly and in a downward direction; this reduces the chances of the runover getting into your eye. Then open your eye and look up, to remove any traces under your lower lashes. Never rub back and forth against your lashes, as this can pull some out and damage the fragile skin on your eyelids.

Next, proceed to your skin cleansing routine. Your cleanser will pick up any remover that remains around your eyes. Close your eyes and rinse them gently by splashing on tepid water with your fingertips. Pat your eyes lightly with a clean towel to dry them.

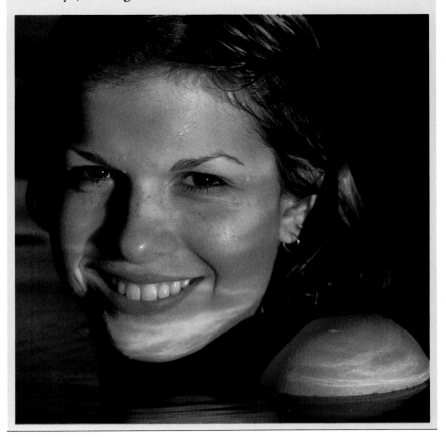

Taking a Closer Look

There is a great amount of potential for enhancing what is unique about your eyes. This inventory is designed to help you identify the specific shape and setting of your eyes, as well as the distance between them, so you can use special makeup techniques to bring out their beauty.

Every woman should be able to experiment with *every* glamour eye makeup technique, not only those dictated by the shape and setting of her eyes. Begin by looking at the illustrations here to find the eyes that most resemble yours in shape or distance from each other. Then read the special tips for adjusting the Glamour Basics eye makeup techniques to match your eyes.

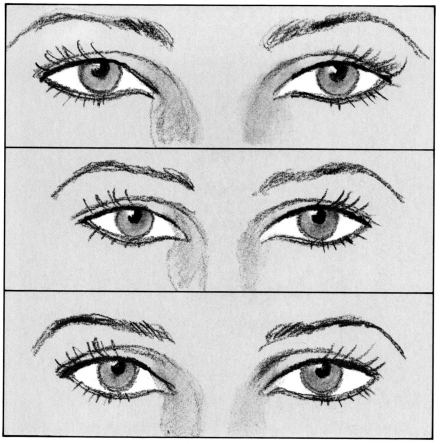

Wide-apart eyes tend to give your face an open, youthful appearance. Intensify this look by applying the strongest eye makeup effects near the outer corners of your eyes. If you wish to make your eyes appear closer together, use more intense eye shadow colors near the inner corners of your eyes.

Close-set eyes can have a dramatic, sultry look that is enhanced by concentrating color near your eyes' inner corners. To make your eyes seem farther apart, apply the most intense color near the outer corners of your eyes.

Evenly spaced eyes are about an eye's distance apart. They can be made to look special with many eye makeup looks. Enhance, dramatize, and define the natural shape of your eyes with the techniques shown here and in the Glamour Adventure.

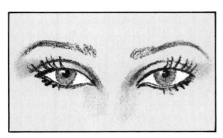

Almond eyes, with their upswept lift at the outer corner, are the most common eye shape. These eyes call for creativity: use color and definition to enhance, shape, and emphasize. Your eyes can look deeper and more intense, innocently open, or as colorful as the rainbow.

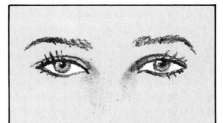

Small eyes are proportionately smaller in comparison to the rest of your facial features. You want these eyes to appear larger and more open — in better balance with your entire face. Light shadow on your eyelids opens up small eyes and gives them greater dimension; more intense shades in the creases help round and enlarge them. Adding lift to the outer corners also opens and widens small eyes; at least two coats of mascara add extra emphasis.

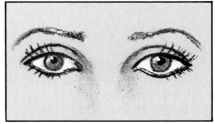

Prominent eyes, set far forward in your face, tend to dominate your facial features. Most often, eyelids are too pronounced. Medium to deep shades. of shadow on the lids help minimize their appearance, and liners applied to your lash bases from corner to corner give prominent eyes a smoldering, mysterious look.

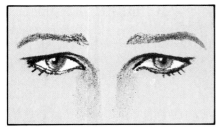

Hooded eyes are set so the natural crease in your eyelid is not readily seen — the upper half of your eyelid dominates. Attention to the crease — with a carefully applied deep, strong shadow color — adds needed dimension and contour to hooded eyes. Highlighting your browbone and lining your lash base gives hooded eyes an alluring shape.

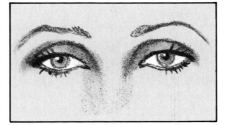

Deep-set eyes, which seem to recede, need to be brought forward. The eyelid crease is set back so the area from the base of your lashes to your browbone seems hidden. Bring out your eyes with a pale shade of eye shadow on your lids that ends just above the hollow of the crease. A neutral eye shadow over the crease emphasizes this area. More intense shading on your browbone also gives your eyes prominence.

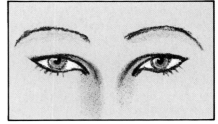

Oriental eyes have a distinctive lift at the outer corner and have very little lid, if any, showing. Deep shades of eye shadow define the crease to add depth, and eyeliner applied as close to the lash base as possible adds dimension. Emphasis on the natural lift at the outer corners of your eyes can play up this feature.

Lip Color
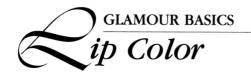

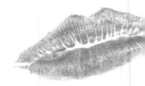

A soft glimmer of lip color harmonizes your whole beautiful look. It is the last step in your basic daytime glamour makeup. Lip color is one of the makeup essentials you should always carry with you. Reapply it often (though never in public). If you have thin lips, or if you drink coffee or smoke regularly during the day, you'll find you need to reapply your lip color more often than normal.

There is a wide range of shades and hues of lip colors from which to choose. When selecting colors consider those complementary (not necessarily perfectly matched) to the color of your clothing and to your cheek and eye colors. First, check the color you've chosen for your cheeks. If you've applied a bright color, select a lip color of equal intensity — perhaps a clear red or a lively pink. If your cheek color is a warm tone, you'll want a lip color in the coral range, possibly with hints of golden peach. In addition, remember that cheek color in the pink range harmonizes with lip color in the rose range; if you choose a strong cheek color to blend with your dark skin, your lip color should be one of the deep russets or spice tones.

Lip color can be more intense than cheek color because the tone is meant not to blend into your skin but to accentuate the shape and contours of your mouth. Avoid lip color that is too strong, however, as it can overpower both your cheek color and eye makeup.

The same color guidelines apply for coordinating lip color with your clothing. Your lip color doesn't have to match them exactly, but it certainly shouldn't clash. The colors should be of the same intensity and range — rosy pinks are best with blues, warm corals and russets go well with clothing in the yellow range, and clear reds look best with both neutrals and primary colors, including red itself.

There are three simple steps to applying lip color, as the illustrations at right show: first, outline and define the shape of your lips with a lip-liner pencil; second, apply a creamy lip color with a lip brush; finally, add the shimmer of lip gloss.

Lip color adds the final polish and balance to your basic daytime glamour makeup. To keep lips fresh with rich, moist color all day long, carry your lining pencil, lip color and application brush, and lip gloss with you whenever you go out.

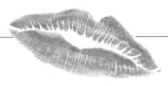

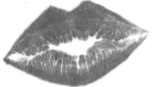

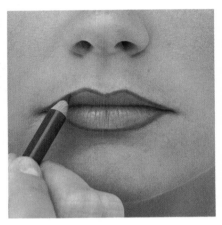

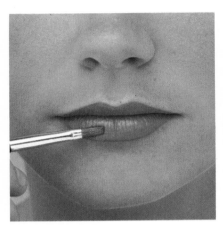

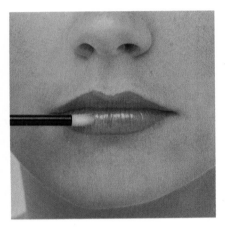

Your **lip-liner** pencil should be slim and have a soft, pointed tip to help you control application. The color of the pencil should complement your lip color — possibly a shade darker. Apply liner pencil carefully, following the natural contours of your mouth to keep your lip color from blurring or bleeding beyond your lips. To apply lip liner, start at the center of your upper lip and draw a fine line out to the corner of your mouth; repeat on the other side. On your lower lip, begin at an outer corner. Finally, use a small, firm-bristled brush to blend the lines outlining your mouth on your lips. (Your lip brush is ideal for blending lip liner.)

To apply creamy **lip color**, stroke your lip brush firmly and evenly across the color. Then, with your mouth relaxed and lips closed, fill in your lips with color. Begin with your upper lip, gently stroking the color from each corner to the center of your mouth so that the lip color is blended into the lip liner. On your bottom lip, begin at one corner of your mouth and sweep the lip color across your lip to the center. Then begin at the other corner and bring the color in to the middle. The color should look rich, radiant, and moist, never heavy or caked.

Lip gloss packaged in a tube with a sponge-tip applicator wand is easiest to use. The best lip glosses add a highly polished shine to your lip color and provide extra moisturizers and sunscreen to protect the delicate skin of your mouth. To use lip gloss, twist the applicator wand slightly in its container so the sponge tip picks up a good amount of gloss. Dot the gloss in the center of your lower lip; the natural movement of your lips will distribute the gloss.

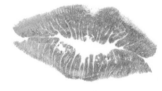

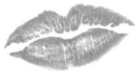

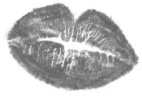

Taking a Closer Look

Your lips should harmonize and balance with your eyes to achieve a complementary and coordinated look. This inventory is designed to help you enhance the appearance of your mouth. As you can see from the illustrations, the variety of lip sizes and shapes is extensive, and although it is almost impossible to change the size or shape of your mouth by applying lip color outside or inside your mouth's natural outline, you can use color to create subtle illusions of improved size and shape.

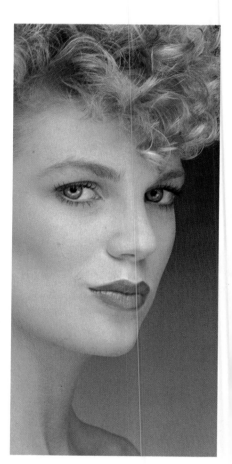

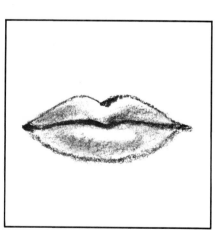

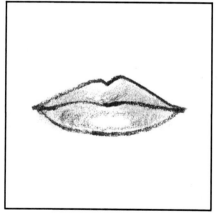

Evenly shaped, **symmetrical lips** are ideally proportioned. They do not need to be reshaped with corrective makeup techniques and are well suited to any number of lip looks.

If you have **asymmetrical lips**, instead of outlining your lips with a lip pencil, use a slightly darker lip color on the larger side of your mouth to balance it with the other side. Blend a darker lip pencil well with this darker lip color to make your lips appear more evenly shaped.

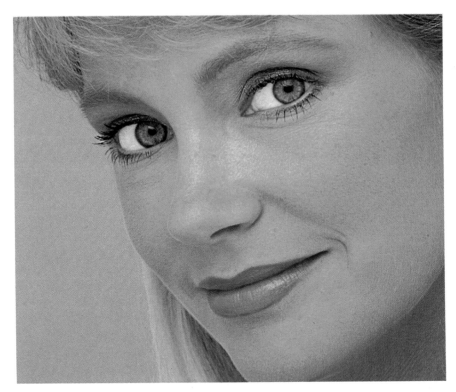

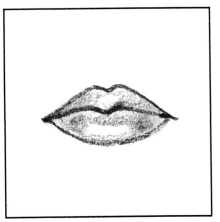

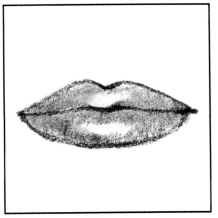

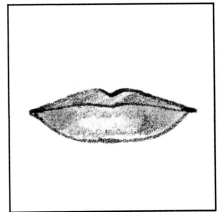

If you have a **_small mouth_**, brighten and dramatize your lips by using an intense shade of lip color and pencil. Select a lip pencil that matches your lip color well. Finish with gloss for extra polish and shine.

Neutral, rather than bright, shades of lip color are most flattering to a **_wide mouth_**. To narrow your lips, try using a darker tone at the corners of your mouth.

When your top and bottom lips are dramatically **_different in size_**, use a light, strong lip color on your smaller lip and a darker, more neutral tone in the same range on the larger one.

Making It Yours

You're looking great — you've learned the daily basics of perfect makeup application that make your cheeks glow with soft color, give subtle definition and shimmering accents to your eyes, and shape and brighten your lips with color. This is the look you want to wear every day, knowing it makes you feel good about yourself. You're confident, groomed, polished, and professional: ready to face the day with the beautiful sense of well-being that comes from looking just right.

And it's so easy to achieve your personal makeup look when you know the best techniques for creating your prettiest face. The Glamour Basics give you a personal system for everyday glamour, a look you can always rely on, a style you can trust to work for you all day long.

Now that you know the basics, why not go even further? Why not extend and expand on what you've learned and take your looks to the limit? Why not aim for the ultimate in dazzling glamour, makeup looks you can wear when your needs go beyond the everyday?

You're now ready to pursue the next level of your beauty potential. You're ready for...

That just-right look of daytime glamour — pretty, polished, and instantly appealing. Knowing you look your best gives you the confidence to face the day — beautifully.

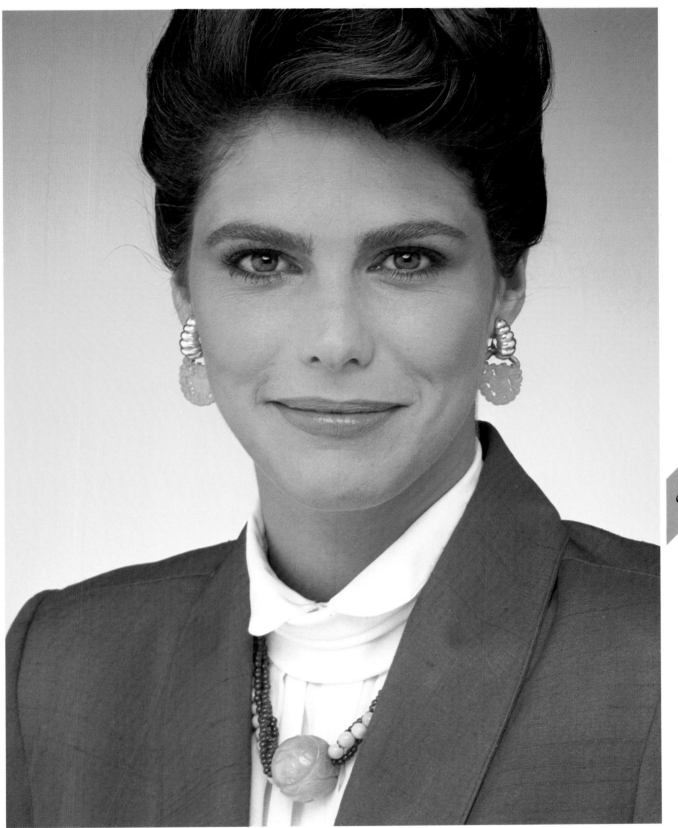

Glamour Adventure

It's an adventure into fabulously exciting makeup techniques, an exploration of your own potential to discover how beautiful you really can be simply by trying what you've never tried before. Go beyond everyday good looks and set your sights on what's different, daring, and dazzling. Take what you've learned from the Glamour Basics and add a sprinkling of sizzle, a dash of drama, a sweep of sophistication, or an exotic flourish of mystery. It's all here — a step-by-step guide to the new beauty discoveries that will take you beyond the basics into the realm of unforgettable glamour magic!

The Glamour Adventure contains more than fifteen different glamour looks that everyone can experiment with, looks designed to help you explore a wonderful variety of cosmetic techniques and colors. The Glamour Adventure will show you new looks to try with that fabulous new dress you just bought or that exciting new haircut you're planning to get. It will teach you new makeup styles for a change in the seasons, a change in your career, or a change in your mood.

Take an hour by yourself or ask a friend to join you in this adventure of new beauty experiments. Try every look — from the most dramatic to the most demure, from the most dynamic to the most spectacularly subtle. And explore your character while you're exploring the potential of your looks. You're sure to discover many delightful surprises — beautiful new ideas that work for you. Be different. Be daring. Be positively dazzling!

Change polish to pizzazz — because a glamour adventure awaits you! Be creative. Experiment. Discover how you can turn a simple daytime look into one that's simply sensational.

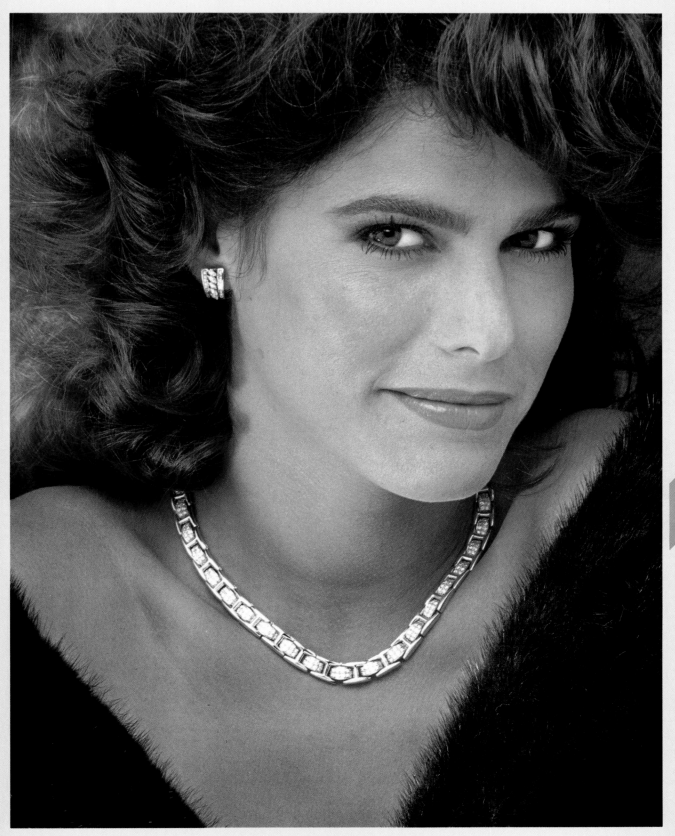

Taking a Closer Look

Makeup is magic. It can change the way you look, both to yourself and to the world. Everyday becomes exciting. Neat becomes a knockout. And simple becomes simply sensational.

The inventory below was designed to get you thinking about the reasons you wear makeup: the way it makes you feel and the effect it has on others. It is also meant to make you think about new ways you can experiment with makeup. You've already seen what basic daytime makeup can do. But why stop there? There are so many opportunities to create enchantment and illusion.

Your answers to the following questions can open your eyes to a Glamour Adventure, an experience in which you can learn how to enhance your best features and be your very own makeup artist.

1. What do you think makeup can do for you?
2. Do you enjoy putting on and experimenting with makeup?
3. Do you wish you knew how to apply makeup better?
4. Do you own a variety of cosmetics?
5. How often do you buy new cosmetics?
6. Before you put on your makeup, do you think about:
   where you are going?
   whom you are going to see?
   what you are going to wear?
   what lighting you are going to be seen in?
   what image you would like to convey?
7. Which of your features do you like best?
8. Which feature do people compliment most often?
9. What colors do you wear to make you feel terrific? (You may want to refer to pages 84 and 85.)

How you feel about makeup most likely reflects how comfortable you are using it and how receptive you are to trying new ideas. Look over your answers, then find the group or groups below that best describe your "makeup personality."

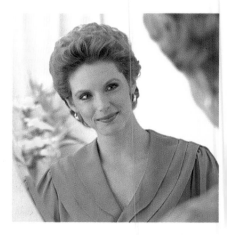

If you're the type who thinks makeup is fun . . . you're probably used to changing your makeup look according to the occasion: where you are going and whom you are going to see. You know how to make your look romantic and feminine, natural and outdoorsy, or daring and bold. For you, makeup expresses a mood and conveys a desired image. Most likely, you own a wide assortment of cosmetics, but that doesn't mean you wouldn't love another new lip or eye color. That's because you enjoy wearing makeup — and it shows.

If you're the type who usually sticks with one basic makeup look . . . maybe it's time to expand your glamour outlook. If you hesitate to vary your look because of your application skills, don't despair. Set aside time to practice with the glamour ideas on the following pages. Or call on a professional beauty consultant for assistance. With some proper guidance and a bit of creativity, you soon will master a wardrobe of makeup styles. And that means you can change your look as often — and as easily — as you change your clothes!

If you're the type who's afraid of looking too "made up" . . . don't be scared off by new ideas. You can look naturally dazzling by controlling the intensity of the colors that you use. (See pages 84 to 87 for more on color and intensity.) Also keep in mind that light has an effect on the balance and tone of color, and that means your makeup can look considerably different depending on the lighting conditions. Because dimmer evening lights can drown out color, your nighttime makeup should be more dramatic and intense. The same holds true for the type of occasion: whereas festive parties call for more daring and adventurous makeup, a candlelight dinner needs a soft and very feminine touch.

If you're the type who will try anything once . . . terrific! The Glamour Adventures on the following pages are tailor-made for you. Try the unexpected: colors you've never worn before, techniques that will give your look a whole new sparkle. Go for the effect — simple and sweet one day, sultry and sophisticated the next. There's no limit to the looks — and images — you can create.

If you're the type who thinks glamour makeup is only for the glamorous . . . it's time to change your thinking. Take note of your best features, the ones you like as well as those others compliment, and learn to enhance them. Take a creative approach to makeup, using ideas from the following pages. Once you become familiar with the techniques, you'll discover how makeup can add a new dimension to your life. And before long, you're likely to find you're among the glamorous, too!

If you find yourself using the same makeup colors . . . you need to experiment with some of the other wonderful shades available. Think about the cheek, eye, and lip colors that you use often because they complement your natural tones. Now check the color chart on page 85 and write down two cheek, eye, and lip colors you've always wanted to try:

Cheek colors _____

_____

Eye colors _____

_____

Lip colors _____

_____

In the pages to come, make a point of experimenting with these colors — and others!

$\mathcal{M}$akeup Tools

To make the most of your Glamour Adventure, be sure you have the following makeup products and tools within easy reach:
- A well-lighted mirror in which you can see yourself clearly; a lighted makeup mirror, which has several different lighting effects, is ideal.
- Cleansing cream, freshener, tissues, cotton, and a clean facecloth dampened with warm water to remove makeup when you want to try the next technique and clean up mistakes you might make while practicing. You'll also need water for your makeup products that need to be mixed with it.
- Cream rouge and several shades of powder blushers, ranging from light to dark, and a blusher blending brush.
- Two highlighter colors with brushes; two basic, or neutral, eye shadow colors with brushes; two darker, or contour, eye shadow colors with brushes; and a clean eye shadow blending brush.
- An eyeliner and mascara in brown or black (whichever suits your coloring) and two eye-defining pencils, one to complement your basic eye shadow colors, the other to complement one of your contour eye shadows. Also, a brow brush and an eyelash brush and curler.
- An assortment of lip colors, one bright, one neutral, and one contrast shade; one lip-liner pencil in a dark shade that blends with your lip colors; and lip gloss. Also, lip brushes for color application and one lip brush for blending.

Chic Cheeks

The makeup accents on your cheeks give shape, structure, softness, and contour to your whole face. It's your first step in makeup, and although it's one of the simplest of techniques, it's also one of the most important. This part of your Glamour Adventure shows you how to experiment with color and contouring to create many exciting glamour looks. As you try these various techniques, you'll see what an enormous difference you can make by applying cheek color in different ways.

You can transform a pretty daytime look into one that's dramatic and dressy by layering three different tones to lift and shape your cheekbones. You can create a soft halo of color that brings out your eyes or sweep color upward to your temples for sensuous sophistication. You can add a bright, sun-kissed glow, a demure youthful blush, or an elegant, high-fashion slant. Cheek color adds instant dazzle and sets the pace for the rest of your makeup.

While you are trying new effects with rouge and blusher, you will also want to experiment with color. Refer to your color inventory, page 85, to find a cheek color you have never used before. Experiment with that — and other — cheek colors in the new ways described on these pages. Experimentation is the key to finding a look that's especially different — and appealing — on you!

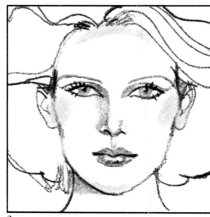

1

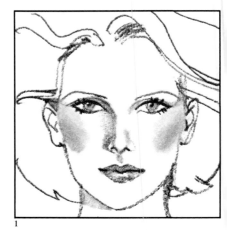

2

1 The Layered Look

You can create a sophisticated look that further dramatizes your cheekbones by skillfully combining three shades of blusher. Follow the procedure on pages 90 and 91 for applying cheek color and contour, then choose a shade slightly darker than your contour color, but in the same color range. Apply the third shade on your outer cheek under the contour shade, on the same level as the bottom of your earlobe. Use a clean blending brush to blend upward and outward so all three shades are well blended with each other. The colors should gradually become more intense as they near your hairline.

2 The Halo Effect

The halo effect adds a very natural all-over glow that brightens your entire face. Using a single shade of blusher — a light or bright shade is best — brush color on your upper cheekbone. Work it down toward the bottom of your earlobe, sweeping it continually outward so that all color starts from the outer corner of your eye. Extend the color onto your earlobes, then lightly brush on color at the top of your forehead, extending it from the arch of one eyebrow to the other. Next, brush a very light curve of blusher across the rounded bottom of your chin.

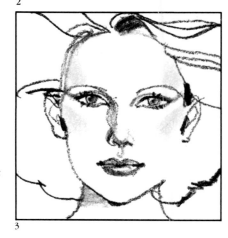

3

118

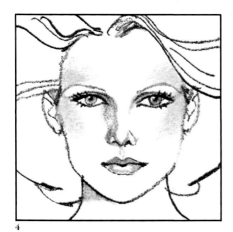

4

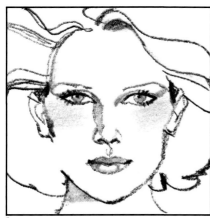

5

3 Sophisticated Diagonals

When blusher is applied in diagonals that sweep dramatically upward, the effect is to thin the face and accentuate its angles, giving a look of glamorous sophistication. Begin by applying color on your cheekbone, where it should be most intense, then brush upward toward your temples. Without adding more color to the brush, bring the color back down, extending it toward the bottom of your nostrils. An upswept diagonal should glow softly across your cheek area. For added lift, apply the same shade of blusher in diagonals above your eyebrows. Begin on your forehead, just above the outer half of your eyebrow, and blend color evenly, up above your temples and out toward your hairline.

4 Color Sweep

An uplifting look that focuses attention on the upper part of your face and on your eyes is created by applying blusher first on your cheekbones, where you want the color to be most intense. Then extend the color up onto your temples, outside the outer corners of your eyes, and up over your eyebrows to the arch points. After applying the blusher so that it forms C-shapes, half encircling your eyes, use a clean blending brush to blend the blusher outward from your cheekbones and temples toward your hairline. Soft, light shades of blusher work best for this look, and blending is very important. Always avoid applying blusher in the immediate eye area.

5 Youthful Blush

Using blusher in a horizontal direction on a face tends to widen the cheekbones and open up the face for a youthful, innocent look. Choose a soft, bright color for this effect, brushing it on the center of your cheeks, beginning at your cheekbone and extending in, to the cheek area below the pupil of your eye. Then, using a blending brush, blend color horizontally, out toward your ear in a straight line.

6 Sunglow

Using blusher to highlight facial areas that are naturally brightened by sunlight creates a glowing, healthy look that softens facial contours. Use a single soft-toned shade of blusher, and begin by applying it first on each cheekbone. Then, without adding more color to your brush, begin with your right cheek and blend color inward, over the bridge of your nose. Repeat from your left cheek, blending color in and over the bridge of your nose. The color should glow over the entire width of your face, from cheekbone to cheekbone. Still without applying more color to your brush, lightly dust the remaining blusher across the center of your forehead, the tip of your chin, and, finally, the tip of your nose.

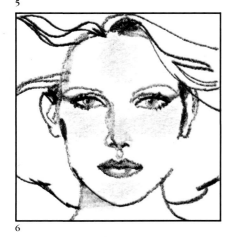

6

Enticing Eyes

There's no denying it — a woman's eyes are her best beauty asset. Admirers focus on eyes that are alive, bright, and rich with splendid color. Eyes that are expressive and memorable. Eyes that make a lasting impression.

The simplest and most dramatic way to enhance your appearance — to add sparkle and excitement to your looks — is to play up your eyes. The skillful application of eye makeup is, in a sense, an art. It's a way to express your feelings, your mood, your sense of style. In the Glamour Adventure for eyes, you'll learn how to use color creatively; how to shape, highlight, line, and define your eyes. And you'll discover dazzling makeup looks for many occasions.

There is a wide range of appealing, eye-catching looks in the Glamour Adventure for eyes — for work and play, for home and evening magic. And you can achieve them all — no matter what size and shape *your* eyes are. All you have to do is read the first instructions, which are for almond-shaped eyes, then follow the variations recommended for your type of eye. (Refer to your eye shape inventory on pages 106 and 107.)

Try the colors suggested here. Or, if you prefer, experiment with your personal favorites. Choose colors to complement your personality, shades to make you look, and feel, sensational. The key is to experiment, to have fun, and to make beautiful eyes a natural part of you. There are no wrong or right looks for anyone, so try them all and take time to get used to the glamorous you they create.

The instructions that follow include three types of eye shadow:
- *Highlighter* — pale and shimmering
- *Basic* — the most classic and neutral
- *Contour* — deep and intense

Before you begin your Glamour Adventure, take a look at the eye shadows in your collection and decide which category each falls into. Also, your choice in both eyeliner and mascara should be compatible with your natural eyelash color, either brown or black. And as a general rule, eye-defining pencils should match the *basic* color of eye shadow used for each look, unless otherwise specified. From there it's up to you. You decide the colors, the combinations, and the intensities that will bring about the glamorous effects you desire!

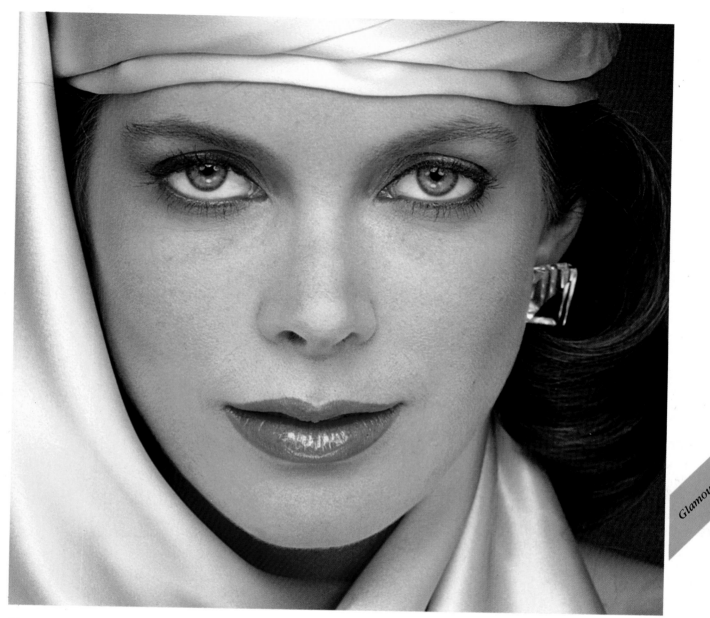

The eyes have it — and here is your chance to be truly creative. Your options are unlimited — be bold and dramatic one day, romantic and feminine the next. You decide. In the Glamour Adventure you'll find eye-appealing looks to suit every mood and occasion.

Angel Eyes

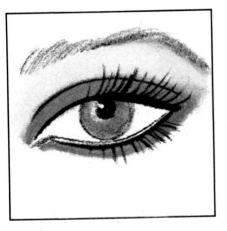

This is a look of soft, glowing color, with naturally highlighted contours, that plays up the sparkle of your eyes. Angel Eyes are for subtle, romantic moods and occasions — sharing a sunset with someone you love, a walk in the country, a casual Sunday brunch, an afternoon picnic. Delicate tones surround your eye with a glimmer of soft highlight on your browbone, giving you a natural, wide-eyed look.

Angel Eyes are created with a basic color and a highlighter, eyeliner, and eye-defining pencil. Here the basic color is plum and the highlighter is ivory.

Step 1: Apply highlighter from your crease up to your eyebrow. *Step 2:* Apply the basic eye shadow color to your eyelid, extending the color up to the crease. *Step 3:* Apply the color around the outer corner of your eye in a narrow line below your lower lashes. *Step 4:* Use a blending brush to blend the basic color into the highlighter. *Step 5:* Apply a thin line of eyeliner above your upper lashes from the inner to the outer corner of your eye. *Step 6:* Apply eye-defining pencil under your lower lashes from the outer to the inner corner of your eye.

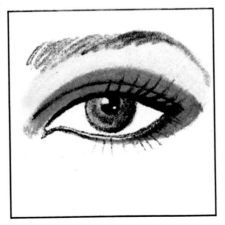

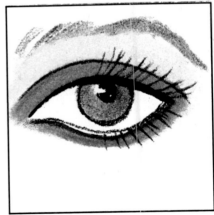

For *small eyes*, extend the color in step 2 slightly above the crease and fan it out at the outer corner of your eye. In step 3, start the color at the outer edge of your iris under the lower lashes and fan the color out to form a soft point with the lid color. In step 5, extend eyeliner slightly beyond the outer corner of your eye. In step 6, begin applying eye-defining pencil slightly beyond the outer corner of your eye and bring the line to the outer edge of your iris.

For *prominent eyes*, apply the basic color in step 3 under your eyes in a thicker line below your lower lashes. In step 5, apply eyeliner a bit more thickly directly above your iris.

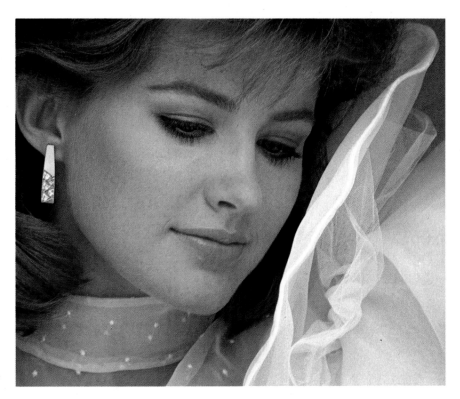

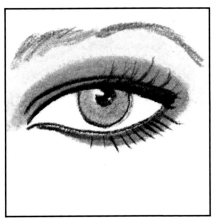

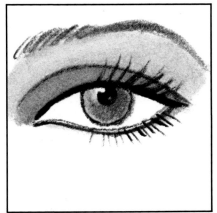

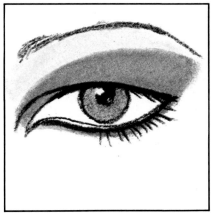

For ***hooded eyes***, emphasize your crease in step 2 by extending the basic eyelid color slightly above the crease. In step 5, apply a thicker line of eyeliner, beginning above the outer edge of your iris and extending to the outer corner of your eye.

For ***deep-set eyes***, apply a darker shade of highlighter in step 1 from your crease up to your eyebrow.

For ***Oriental eyes***, apply the basic color in step 2, beginning at the inner corner of your eyelid and fanning the color up toward the outer end of your brow.

Muted Doe Eyes

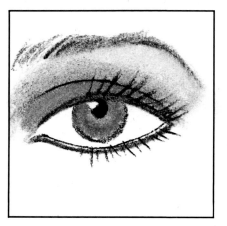

Muted Doe Eyes are dramatic and smoky, a harmoniously blended glimmer of three eye shadow tones to imitate the beguiling beauty of a deer's round eye. This look hints at the sophistication and sultry mood of candlelit dinners or moonlit strolls. These eyes glow with anticipation and glisten with mystery. Eye shadow tones halo the eye with muted colors — here, green, brown, and pale almond.

Muted Doe Eyes are created with highlighter, basic color, and contour, and with eyeliner and eye-defining pencil. Your choice of shades can go from delicately subtle (for an evening for two) to deeply intense (for an elegant party).

Step 1: Apply highlighter from your crease up to your eyebrow. *Step 2:* Apply the basic color to your eyelid, extending the color up to the crease. *Step 3:* Apply contour color in the crease, slightly tapering the color as you extend it from the inner to the outer corner. *Step 4:* Use a blending brush to blend the highlighter and the basic color into the contour color. *Step 5:* Apply a thin line of eyeliner above your upper lashes from the inner to the outer corner of your eye. *Step 6:* Apply eye-defining pencil (in the same color as the contour color) under your lower lashes from the outer to the inner corner of your eye.

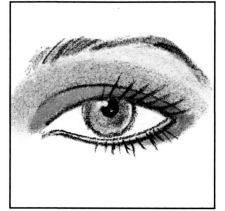

For **small eyes**, extend the basic color in step 2 beyond the outer corner of your eye. Then bring the color down below your lower lashes to form a soft point at the outside corner. In step 3, apply the contour color in the inner underbrow area, extending it up to your eyebrow.

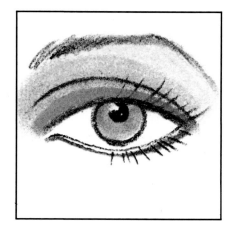

For **prominent eyes**, apply the basic color in step 2 on your eyelid halfway up to the crease. Apply the contour color in step 3 upward from the basic color. In step 6, apply a slightly thicker line of eye-defining pencil under your lower lashes from the outer to the inner corner.

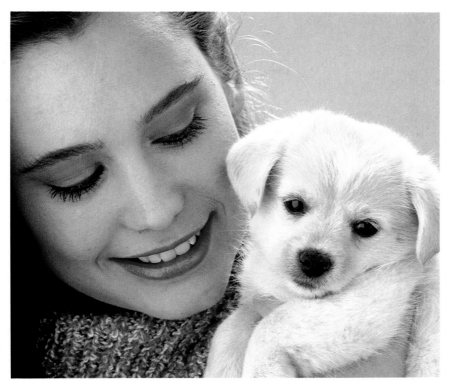

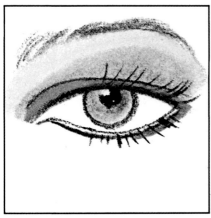

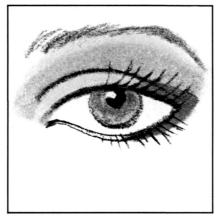

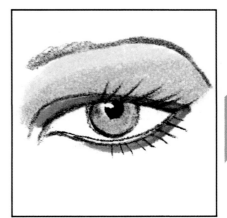

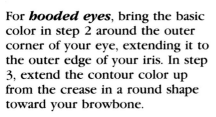

For ***hooded eyes***, bring the basic color in step 2 around the outer corner of your eye, extending it to the outer edge of your iris. In step 3, extend the contour color up from the crease in a round shape toward your browbone.

For ***deep-set eyes***, apply highlighter in step 1 just under your brow and on your eyelid from the inner corner of your eye to the outer edge of your iris. In step 2, apply the basic color from the outer edge of your iris to just beyond the outer corner of your eye. Then extend the color below your lower lashes to the outer edge of your iris. Extend the contour color in step 3 up from the crease and fan it out toward the outer edge of your eyebrow.

For ***Oriental eyes***, extend the basic color in step 2 under your lower lashes from the outer corner of your eye to the inner edge of your iris. In step 3, apply the contour color, beginning at the inner corner of your eye above the crease and fanning it out to the outer brow.

Starlit Eyes

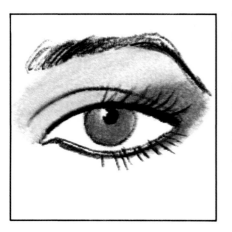

This eye holds mystique and magic, the shimmer of starlight, the mood of a midnight sky. Starlit Eyes are for elegant dresses, dancing till dawn, glittering parties, and late suppers in town. The look is upswept, the hues intense, the contours dramatic. These eyes are for evening, for making an impression on everyone or one special someone.

The Starlit Eye is created with highlighter and contour color; here, the highlighter is silver-blue and the contour is deep gray-blue.

Step 1: Apply highlighter over your entire eyelid, from your upper lashes to your eyebrow. *Step 2:* Beginning above the center of your pupil, apply the contour color in a wedge shape, fanning the color out from the middle of your lid up to your brow. *Step 3:* Bring the contour color around the outer corner of your eye, under your lashes, to the outer edge of your iris. *Step 4:* Using a blending brush, blend the contour color upward and outward into the highlighter. *Step 5:* Apply a thin line of eyeliner above your upper lashes from the inner to the outer corner of your eye. *Step 6:* Apply eye-defining pencil under your lower lashes from the outer to the inner corner of your eye.

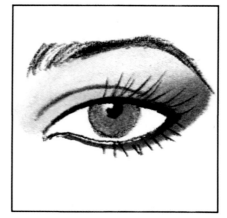

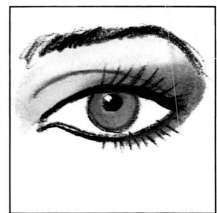

For **small eyes**, begin applying contour color in step 2 at the outer edge of your iris, forming a wedge at the outer corner of your eye. In step 3, bring the contour color around the outer corner, under your lower lashes, to the middle of your eye. In step 5, apply eyeliner slightly more thickly at the outer corner.

For **prominent eyes**, begin applying contour color in step 2 at the inner edge of your iris and fan the color out toward the outer edge of the brow. In step 3, bring the contour color down under your lower lashes to the middle of your eye.

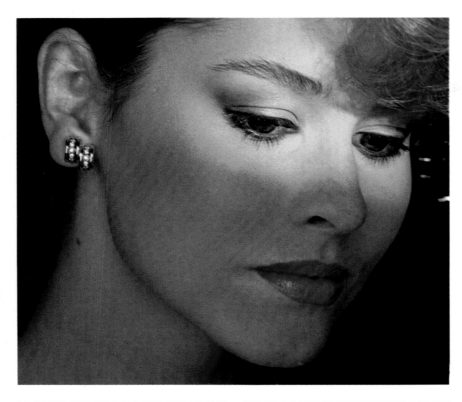

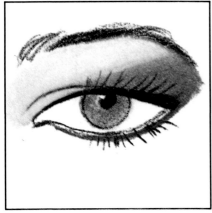

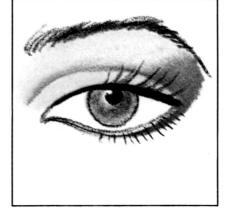

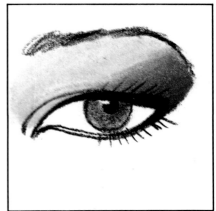

For **_hooded eyes_**, apply the contour color in step 2 beginning at the inner edge of your iris, then fan the color upward and outward to the brow. When applying contour color under your lower lashes in step 3, extend it inward in a fine line to the middle of your eye.

For **_deep-set eyes_**, apply highlighter more heavily over the entire lid and brow area. In step 2, apply contour color outward from the crease to the brow, beginning at the outer edge of your iris. In step 3, extend the contour color under your lower lashes in a fine line to the outer edge of your iris.

For **_Oriental eyes_**, apply the contour color in step 2 in a wedge shape from the inner edge of your iris, fanning outward and upward to the outer edge of your brow. When applying eyeliner in step 5, make the line slightly thicker from the inner edge of the iris to the outer corner of the eye. Extend the line just around the outer corner of your eye to form a wedge.

ᗡazzle Eyes

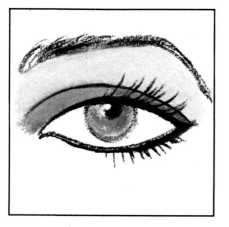

This multishaded, multifaceted look draws all eyes to you. Dazzle Eyes cast a spell; they're luxurious, bewitching, unforgettable. The mood of this eye is romantic, sophisticated, intensely dramatic. Dazzle Eyes are for the seductive glance, the flirtatious wink, the exotic mood — an evening shared by the fire, a party on a penthouse terrace, elegant restaurants. Dazzle Eyes express chameleon changes; their glances are sought and held. They're daring, exciting, and always noticed.

This look lets you explore your eye shadow palette, using three different hues for dramatic dazzle; here the highlighter is ivory, the basic color is rosy plum, and the contour is midnight blue.

Step 1: Apply highlighter from your crease up to your eyebrow. *Step 2:* Apply the basic color on your eyelid up to the crease from the inner corner of your eye to the center of your pupil. *Step 3:* Apply the contour color on the outer half of your eyelid. Blend the shadows well with a blending brush. *Step 4:* Apply a fine line of eyeliner above your upper lashes from the inner to the outer corner of your eye. *Step 5:* Apply eye-defining pencil (in the same color as the basic color) under your lower lashes from the outer corner of your eye to the outer edge of your iris.

For ***small eyes***, extend the basic color in step 2 slightly above the crease. Apply the contour color in step 3 slightly above the crease. Then bring it down around the outer corner of your eye, under your lashes, to the middle of your eye. The color should form a wedge just above the outer corner, tapering upward to the outer brow. In step 5, apply a slightly thicker line of eyeliner from the outer edge of your iris to the outer corner of your eye.

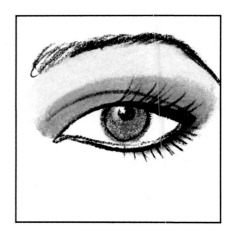

For ***prominent eyes***, bring the contour color in step 3 down around the outer corner of your eye, under your lashes, and extend it to the inner edge of your iris. In step 5, apply a thicker line of eyeliner above your upper lashes, bringing the eyeliner slightly around and under the outer corner of your eye.

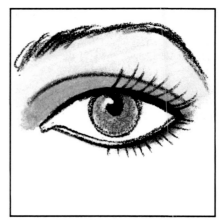

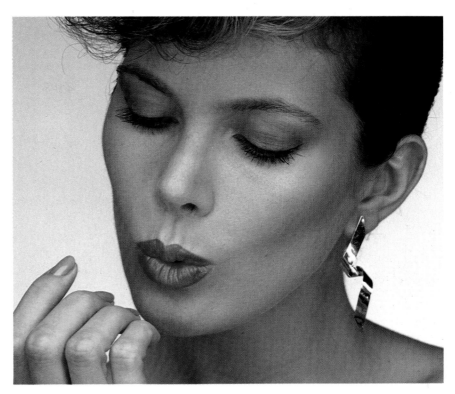

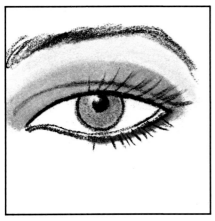

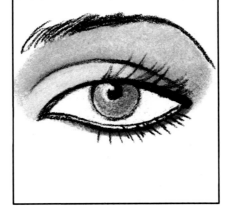

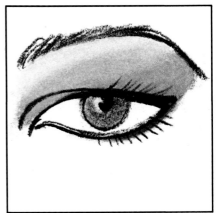

For ***hooded eyes***, extend the basic color in step 2 slightly above the crease. Also extend the contour color in step 3 slightly above the crease to just beyond the outer corner, then down under your lower lashes in a thin line to the middle of your eye.

For ***deep-set eyes***, apply highlighter on your eyelid in step 2, instead of the basic color, from the inner corner of your eye to the outer edge of your iris. Apply the basic color from the crease up to your eyebrow. In step 3, apply a thin line of the contour color under your lower lashes from the outer corner of your eye to the outer edge of your iris. In step 6, use a cotton swab to smudge eye-defining pencil from the outer to the inner corner of your eye.

For ***Oriental eyes***, extend the basic color in step 2 from the inner corner of your eye upward and outward to your eyebrow. In step 3, fan the contour color from the inner edge of your iris out to your eyebrow to form a wedge. Bring contour color under your lower lashes from the outer corner to the middle of your eye. In step 4, extend liner beyond the outer corner of your eye in a wedge. In step 5, apply a thicker line of eye-defining pencil to the middle of your eye.

Rainbow Eyes

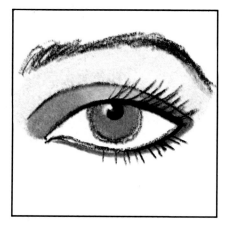

These eyes radiate a gentle glow of four different eye shadow colors, a medley of blended tones that gives off the elusive shimmer of a rainbow. The look is vivid, striking, spectacular, and never shy: always the center of attention. The mood is strictly main event — to match your most stunning gown, your most glamorous hairdo, your most fashionable mood. These Cinderella eyes take you to the ball.

Rainbow Eyes exalt every aspect of your own beautiful eyes; they're created with two highlighters, a basic color, and a contour. Here, the lighter shade of highlighter is ivory and the darker, almond. The basic shade is soft violet and the contour, moss green.

Step 1: Apply the lighter shade of highlighter from your crease up to your eyebrow. *Step 2:* Apply the darker shade of highlighter on the middle third of your eyelid (from the inner to the outer edge of your iris), up to the crease. *Step 3:* Apply the basic color on the inner third of your eyelid, up to the crease. *Step 4:* Apply the contour color on the outer third of your lid, up to the crease. *Step 5:* Blend all shadows with a blending brush. *Step 6:* Apply a thin line of eyeliner above your upper lashes from the inner to the outer corner of your eye. *Step 7:* Apply eye-defining pencil under your lower lashes from just beyond the outer corner to the inner corner of your eye. Smudge the color with a cotton swab to soften and thicken the line.

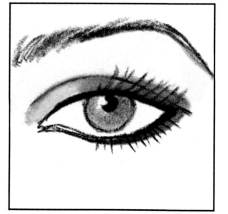

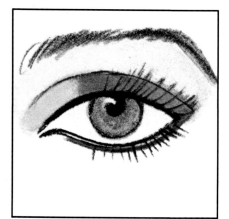

For **small eyes**, apply the darker shade of highlighter on the inner third of your eyelid and the basic color on the middle third. In step 4, extend the contour color slightly above the crease and just beyond the outer corner of your eye. Also extend the eyeliner in step 6 just beyond the outer corner of your eye to form a wedge. In step 7, apply eye-defining pencil slightly more thickly at the outer corner.

For **prominent eyes**, apply the darker shade of highlighter on the inner third of your lid, the contour color on the middle third, and the basic color on the outer third. In step 6, apply eyeliner slightly more thickly above the pupil. In step 7, eye-defining pencil should be applied slightly more thickly below the pupil.

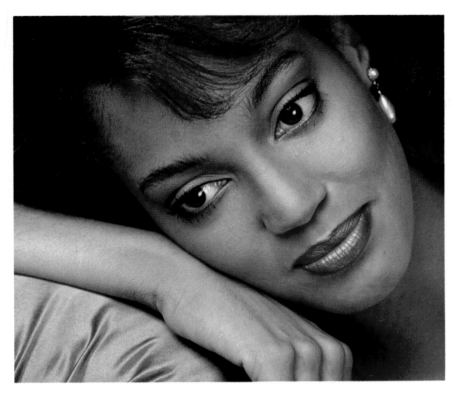

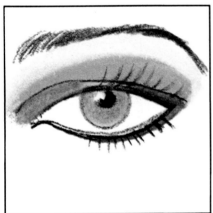

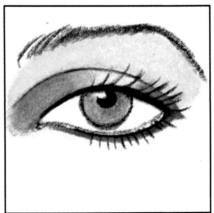

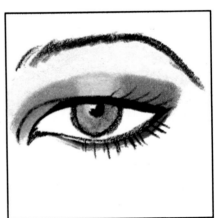

For ***hooded eyes***, apply a second contour shade to your crease in step 4; a neutral shade, such as brown or gray, is best.

For ***deep-set eyes***, apply the darker rather than lighter shade of highlighter in step 1 from the crease to the eyebrow. Apply the lighter shade of highlighter on the middle third of your lid, the basic color on the inner third, and the contour color on the outer third.

For ***Oriental eyes***, extend the eye shadow colors in steps 2, 3, and 4 over the crease, halfway up to your eyebrow. Extend the contour color slightly upward toward your brow.

Luscious Lips

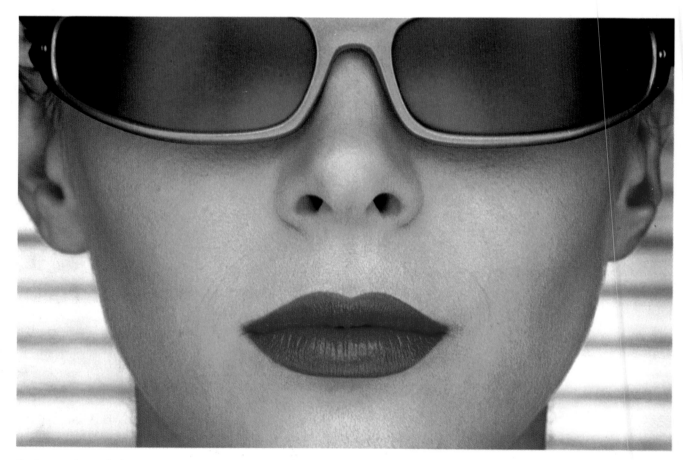

Deliciously rich lips, dressed in glorious, spirited color: because so much of your inner beauty and feelings are conveyed in your smile, you want lip color that's clear, fresh, and vibrant. It's easy to see why lips are the important finale to every great glamour look.

No matter what your mood — flirty or feminine, daring or dazzling, playful or professional — you'll find a lip look to match. The effects illustrated on the following pages will not only balance out any makeup style, they'll add an unmistakable sparkle to your smile.

Begin by referring to your inventory of glamour (see pages 116 and 117), to recall a lip color you want to try. Experiment with the different intensities of every color to find the one that works wonderfully for you.

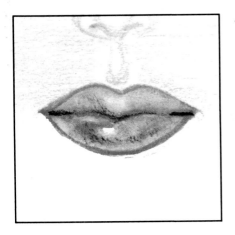

Shimmer Lips

When your mood is subtle and your look natural, Shimmer Lips will add a bare tint of color and lots of shine. These lips are nothing less than irresistible. Begin by outlining your lips with your lip-liner pencil, carefully following their exact shape. Then use your clean lip brush to blend the pencil outline onto your lips. The color should be very pale, with a slightly darker outline. Next, dot lip gloss on the center of each lip and distribute the gloss with the same lip brush, which will still have some lip pencil color on it. Press your lips gently together to blend color and gloss.

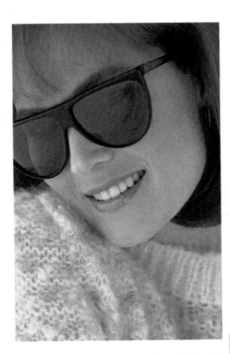

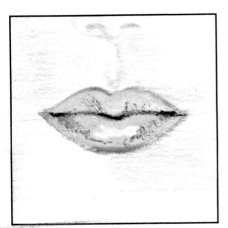

Color-Kissed Lips

Color-Kissed Lips make your mouth glow with natural color; the warm color looks as though it comes from within, like ripening fresh berries or a flowering rose. The effect is seductively innocent and utterly kissable. Outline your lips with lip-liner pencil, then brush on your choice of lip color. Gently press your lips together to distribute color evenly, then blot them firmly on a tissue. Continue blotting on different parts of a clean tissue until only the palest color shows. Now apply a dot of lip gloss to the center of each lip. Wipe excess lip color from your lip brush and use it to distribute the gloss over both lips. Press your lips gently together to distribute gloss and color.

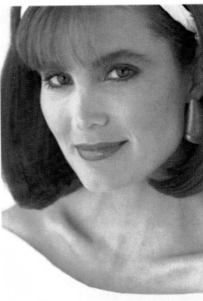

Luscious Lips

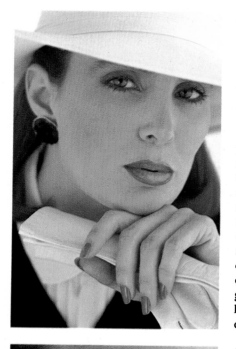

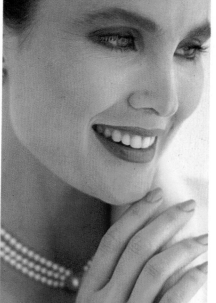

Pucker-Up Lips

This look narrows the width of your mouth into a pretty pucker, a kiss of color that draws attention to the central shape of your lips. These lips have a sense of fun. Begin by outlining your lips with a lip-liner pencil one shade darker than your lip color. Then use the pencil to fill in the darker shade from the corners of your mouth toward the center, so that the darker shade stops on a line with the outer edge of your nostrils. Blend well with a clean lip brush and apply lip color to the central area of your mouth. Also blend lip color into the lip pencil at the outer corners. Apply a dot of lip gloss to the center of your bottom lip. Press lips gently together to distribute gloss and color evenly.

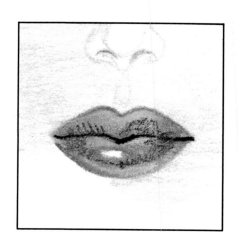

Hot Lips

When cheeks are made up to be intensely sophisticated and eyes mysteriously smoldering, Hot Lips give your mouth the same dimension of elegance and mystique. The look brings your mouth forward to give added attention to a graceful curve of jaw, a pretty chin, your whole lower face. This is a look for those times you want your lips to be *noticed.* Begin by gently patting white highlighter foundation (see page 73) around the skin above your upper lip, blending well. Next, use a contour shade of blusher with a small brush high on your chin, just under the slight pout at the center of your bottom lip, forming a well-blended, horizontal line right below your bottom lip. Apply lip-liner pencil,

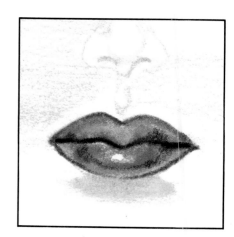

blending it with a lip brush; follow with lip color and a dot of gloss to your bottom lip. Press your lips gently together to distribute the gloss and color.

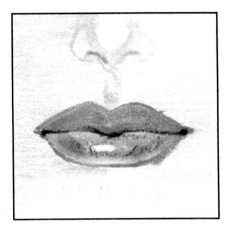

Pouty Mouth

A bright and/or light shade of lip color on your bottom lip gives it flirtatious prominence to create a mischievously sultry pout. The Pouty Mouth is youthfully romantic, whimsical, and festive. Use the same color lip pencil on top and bottom lips. Blend the pencil line on your lips, then fill in the top lip with color and the bottom lip with a lighter shade in the same color range. Add a dot of gloss in the center of the bottom lip. Don't press your lips together, or you'll blend the two shades and diminish the effect.

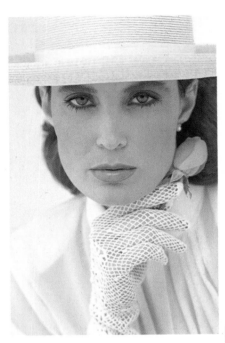

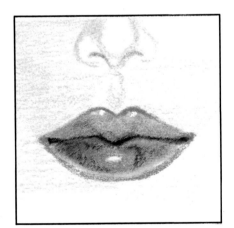

Cupid's Bow

Accentuating your top lip with added contour gives your mouth sheer feminine prettiness — a look that is all ruffles, lace, and roses. Using a lip-liner pencil that matches your lip color, outline your lips, giving the two upward curves of your top lip emphasis by slightly exaggerating their rounded points. (But keep them in line with your nostrils and even with each other.) Blend the lip pencil with your lip brush. Then use a light shade of lip color on your upper lip and a neutral, darker shade on your lower lip. Dot lip gloss just below each point on your upper lip and in the center of your lower lip. Don't press your lips together, or you'll blend the two shades.

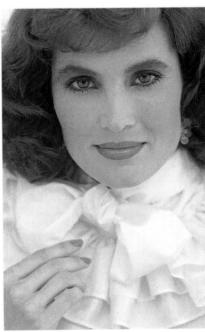

135

Putting It All Together

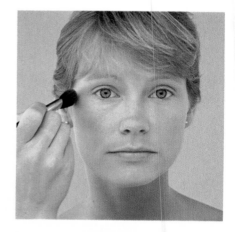

Soft, natural, and country casual are the words that best sum up what Kate requires from a makeup look. She runs a part-time business with her husband from their rural home, and because she deals with customers every day she has to look her best. At the same time, Kate's country setting calls for a natural look that's never overdone. In addition to managing her business Kate is the mother of a toddler and has a fairly tight schedule every day.

For cheeks, Kate chooses the Sunglow effect from the Glamour Adventure in a soft pink tone; the pink brightens her light skin coloring by adding a subtle contrast to her golden tones.

In the morning, after applying basic foundation, Kate brushes her blusher on the tops of her cheekbones and over the bridge of her nose; next, she lightly dots some color on her nose, chin, and upper forehead. The result — a fresh, youthful, all-over blush that suits her casual style perfectly.

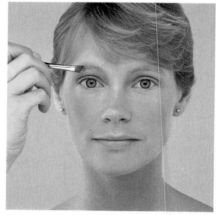

For eyes, Kate wants the soft glow of color she gets from the Angel Eyes in the Glamour Adventure. To complement her own eye color, she applies blue as the basic eye shadow color on her lid and an almond highlighter on her browbone and inner underbrow area. She brings the blue shadow down under her eye on her lower lash base, and intensifies the color by using a blue eye-defining pencil before sweeping on brown mascara.

For lips, Kate wants the bare hint of color she achieves with the Shimmer Lips look for the Glamour Adventure. She outlines her lips with a lip-liner pencil in a deep tone and blends the color on her lips with a lip brush. Then Kate dots on gloss and blends again.

The complete look takes only a few minutes each day and is just what Kate needs from her makeup — warm and polished, with a few bright touches that make her best features stand out.

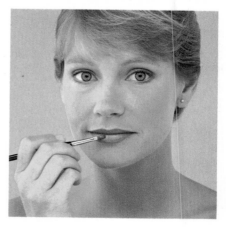

For a look that's soft and polished, Kate keeps her beauty routine simple. In just a few minutes a day, she can achieve the natural, well-groomed appearance her busy lifestyle demands.

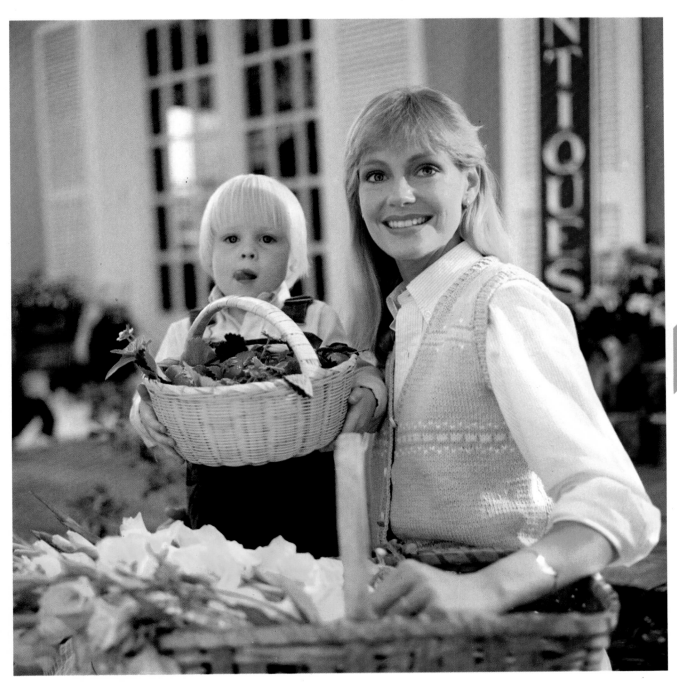

Putting It All Together

June needs a sophisticated daytime look for her career in cosmetics sales. She wants to project an image of glamour and elegance with her daily makeup because she sets beauty standards for the people she works with. June and her husband also entertain frequently, and since she often doesn't have time for more than freshening her daytime makeup in the evening, June needs a makeup look that takes her straight from a busy day into a social evening.

June adds emphasis to the lovely angles of her cheekbones by using diagonal strokes of color on them, as well as above her brows. She begins with clear red cream cheek color, followed by a soft berry blusher. For a final touch of color, she applies what's left of the blusher on her brush in diagonals over her eyebrows, from the center arch point of each brow upward and outward toward her upper temples, creating the Sophisticated Diagonals look from the Glamour Adventure. This look goes from day to night with just a touch of a darker blusher shade applied over her daytime color.

For eyes, June uses the dramatic Rainbow Eye look from the Glamour Adventure, softened for day with a subtle choice of eye shadow colors — violet on the inner corner of her lid, pale blue highlighter on the center of her lid, and midnight blue on the outer corner of her eyelid, extended up and out at the outer corner of her eye to emphasize the natural uplift of her eyes, and brought below her eye to the lower lash base for surrounding glow. A shimmer of ivory highlighter on her browbone and inner underbrow area is blended well down into the eyelid colors. For evenings, June accentuates her eyes by adding a fine line of black eyeliner on her upper lash base and a line of misty violet eye-defining pencil under her lower lash base. An extra touch of mascara adds elegance.

For lips, June chooses the Hot Lips mouth to balance her dramatic eyes. She applies highlighter foundation on the skin above her top lip, then wisps on a contour shade of berry blusher just under her lower lip, using a small brush to form a horizontal line under the slight pout of this lip. She outlines both lips in a deep-toned lip-liner pencil, then fills them in with deep coral lip color. The final touch is a dot of lip gloss on the center of her lower lip.

The complete look offers June the kind of fashionable sophistication she needs for her career every day and, with a few touches, allows her to be ready in a few minutes for social evenings.

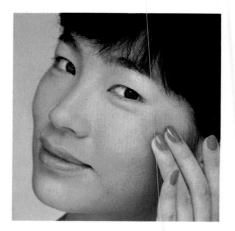

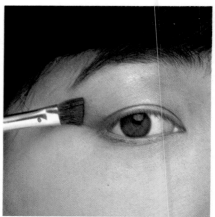

With a career in cosmetic sales and an active social schedule, June needs a makeup look that's sophisticated and long-lasting. She chooses colors and application techniques that take her from day to evening.

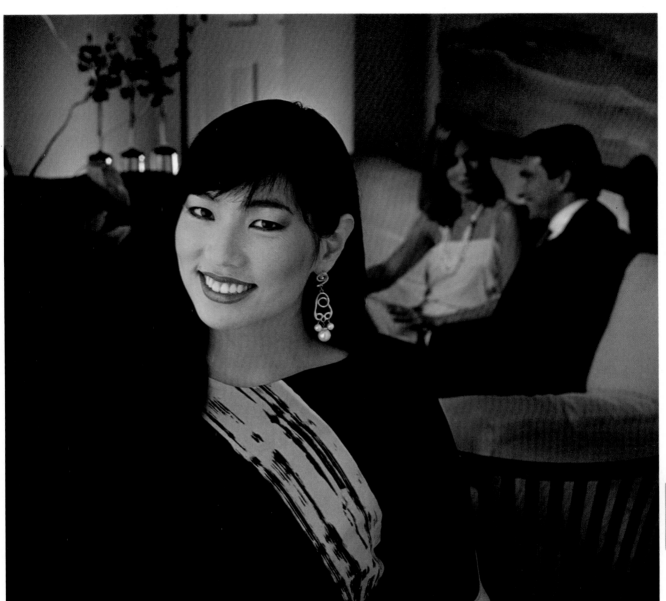

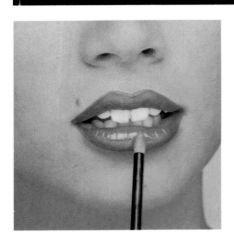

Putting It All Together

Meg has a busy professional city life with an active evening social schedule. She requires makeup that gives her a serious working woman image for day and a sophisticated, elegant style for night.

Meg applies a red cream cheek color, which she follows with soft berry blusher over her cheekbones for a workday look. To add sophistication for evening, Meg applies a deeper berry shade of blusher in the hollows of her cheeks below her cheekbones and daytime cheek color. The second cheek color instantly takes Meg's look from basic daytime polish to evening dazzle.

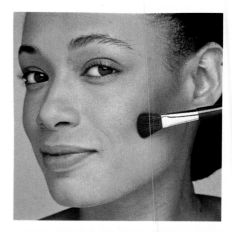

For eyes, Meg uses the Glamour Basics look on the job — plum eye shadow on her lid and almond highlighter on her browbone and inner underbrow area. A fine line of black eyeliner on her upper lash base and black mascara on her lashes complete her professional daytime look. To glamorize her workday eyes, Meg adds touches required for the Muted Doe Eyes in the Glamour Adventure. She takes the plum eye shadow on her lid down under her eye to the lower lash base, then strengthens the color by adding a light line of misty violet eye-defining pencil. She touches up her almond highlighter, adding more color to her browbone to accentuate the contour of her eyes, then applies a deep brown eye shadow to the crease of her eye to give it depth. An extra application of black mascara darkens and thickens her lashes.

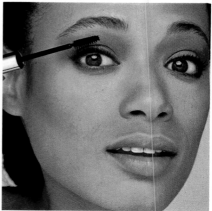

For lips, Meg uses the technique from Glamour Basics — lip-liner pencil to outline her lips in a red tone, filled in with a medium red lip color and finished with a touch of lip gloss. When she's going out at night, Meg freshens her lip color with flourishes of the Cupid's Bow Mouth from the Glamour Adventure; she outlines her lips in a red-toned lip-liner pencil, accentuating the two points on her upper lip; then she applies a deep rose lip color and lip gloss.

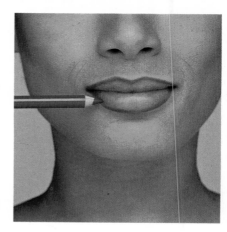

Meg's complete look projects exactly the image she wants to create — for day, the subtle luster of attractive, straightforward makeup; for evening, the touches of glamour that add instant panache. Once she achieves her basic look — the polish of a professional woman — she can quickly convert it to dazzle at the end of her workday.

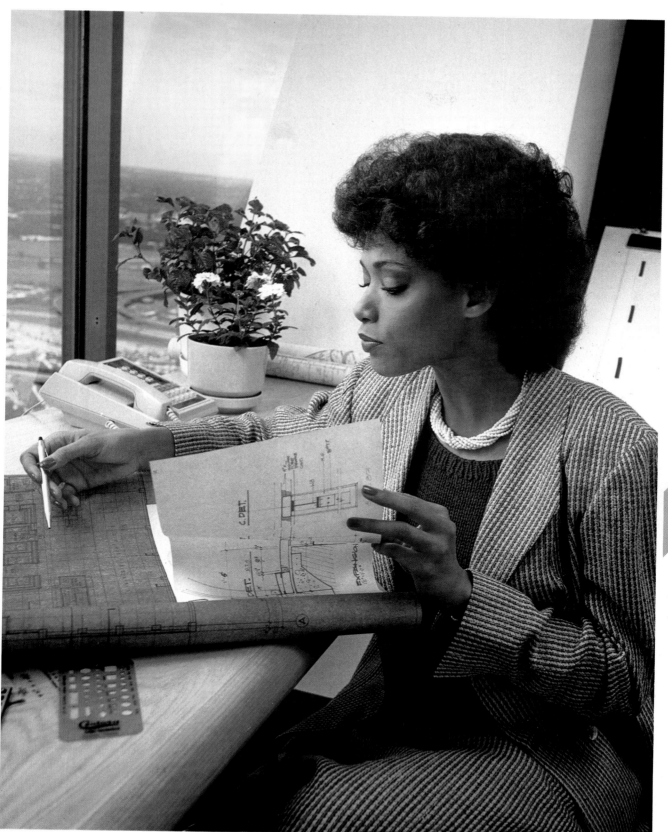

141

FOUR

Hair Care

Hair that's everything it should be — soft, shining, healthy, and full of life. Taking care of your hair means keeping it clean and conditioned, choosing a style that complements you and fits in with the details of your beauty program. Your hairstyle — short or long, curly or straight — showcases your features and expresses the importance you place on looking your very best. Because your beautiful hair literally shimmers with health, vitality, and personal style.

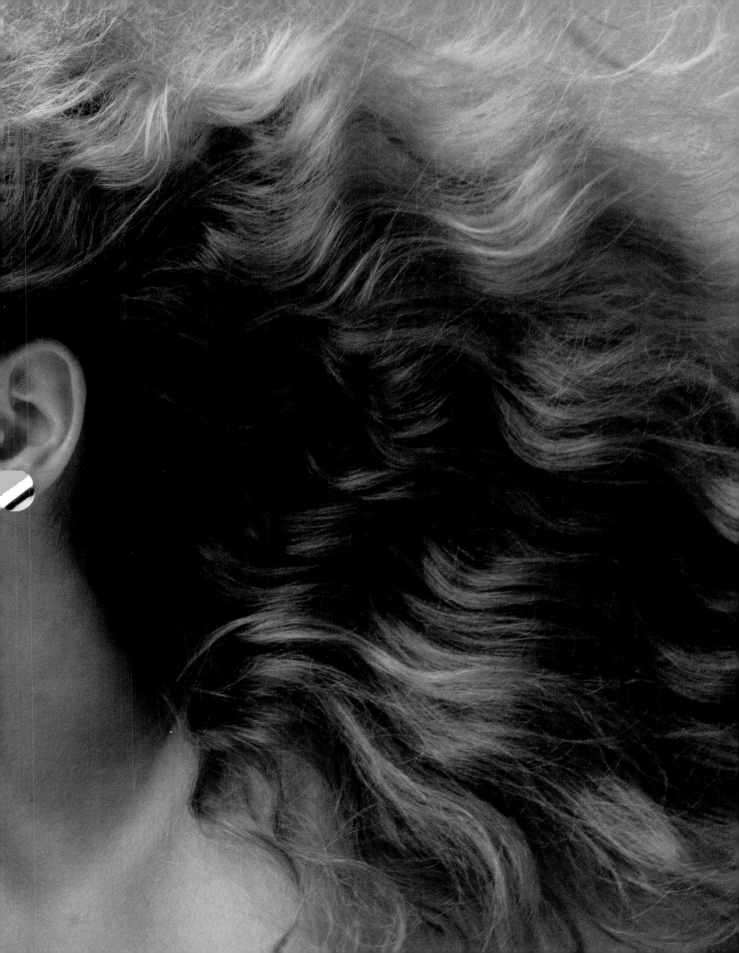

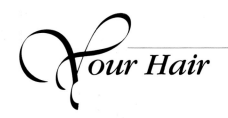

Your Hair

Most people take their hair for granted, assuming that if they wash it regularly, it will stay beautiful and healthy. But there's more to beautiful hair than just shampoo and water. To care for your hair properly you should have a basic knowledge of its functions — the factors that contribute to its condition and texture, the amount of hair you have, and its color.

The hair on your scalp is similar to the epidermis, or outer layer, of your skin. Hair is made of dead cells pushed upward by new living cells in the hair follicle. Like the skin's surface, the cells that make up a strand of hair contain the protein keratin. Between one hundred thousand and two hundred thousand hair follicles produce the hair strands on your scalp. Oil (sebaceous) glands attached to the hair follicles produce and secrete the oily substance sebum, which lubricates and smooths the hair strands as they move upward toward the surface.

The average growth rate of hair is approximately one-half inch each month, or six inches a year. After a growing period of four to ten years, the root of each hair goes into a resting period of about three months, during which the base of the hair follicle shrinks and no new cells are produced. At the end of the rest period, hair cells begin to multiply again, pushing new strands of hair toward the scalp's surface and causing the "old" hair to loosen and fall out. As a result it isn't unusual to experience some hair loss daily. (The cycles of growth and rest occur on different schedules all over the scalp so that no one area is losing all its hair at the same time.) Only five thousand to ten thousand hair follicles, scattered over the head, are dormant at any given time.

The texture of your hair is determined by the diameter of each strand of hair. A strand of coarse hair is relatively large in diameter, while a strand of fine hair is relatively small in diameter. If your hair is very thick you probably have a great many hair follicles; if your hair is thin you have a smaller number of hair follicles. The number of hair follicles you have and the size of individual hair strands are basically factors of heredity, although proper conditioning and styling techniques can help correct extremes.

The cross-sectional shape of each strand is what makes hair straight, wavy, or curly: perfectly round strands produce straight hair; flat, oval-shaped hair shafts produce wavy hair; and very curly

A cross section of a strand of growing hair illustrates its structure. Each hair follicle has an arrector pili muscle attached to it. When cold or fear makes the muscles contract, your hair stands straight up and your scalp gets goose bumps.

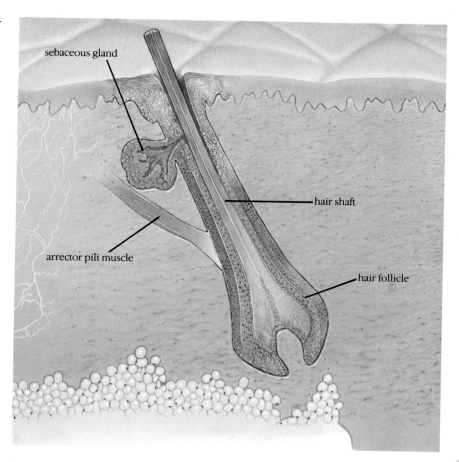

sebaceous gland

hair shaft

arrector pili muscle

hair follicle

hair is composed of flatter, kidney-shaped strands. This is another genetically determined characteristic of hair.

The color of your hair is governed by melanin, the same pigment that gives color to your skin. Less melanin may be produced as you get older, causing hair to gray.

Your hair can become one of your most versatile and important beauty assets. Whether you wear it long or short, curly or straight, your hair is one of the first things people notice about you. And when you decide to change your cut or style, you know your hair will continue to grow and renew itself constantly. So whatever your preferences in hairstyles, it's essential that you maintain a healthy routine of hair care.

Taking a Closer Look

Every woman wants her hair to be healthy and lustrous, to shine and have lots of bounce. She also wants a flattering hairstyle that is easy to care for. A basic hair-care system lays the groundwork for all these goals. To care for your hair properly, however, you must first understand its characteristics: quantity, type, texture, overall condition, and even the shape and size of each individual hair strand.

The following inventory is designed to help you determine the nature of your hair. Complete the statements below as accurately as possible by evaluating the characteristics of your hair at the present time. If you color your hair, have a permanent, or treat it chemically in any way, circle the appropriate answer with respect to your hair's current condition, rather than its natural state.

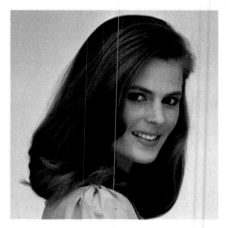

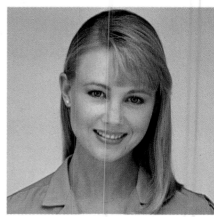

The woman at the top has a head of thick hair, whereas the woman in the lower photo is an example of someone with thin hair.

1. **Twenty-four to forty-eight hours after shampooing, regardless of the products I use, my hair:**
   A. Looks and feels better than it does right after shampooing, when it tends to be dull and flyaway.
   B. Does not look or feel significantly different from the way it does right after shampooing.
   C. Feels matted down and greasy; it sticks together in clumps and looks darker at the roots.

2. **My hair generally responds to the cold, dry winter climate and the hot, damp summer climate in the following manner:**
   A. In the winter, my hair becomes very dry and flyaway and often has static electricity; in the summer, my hair seems more stabilized and easier to control.
   B. In the winter, my hair tends to become dry and sometimes has static electricity; in the summer, my hair tends to become slightly oily and limp.
   C. In the winter, my hair seems more normal and I seldom have problems with flyaway hair or static electricity; in the summer, my hair becomes oily and limp and seems to get dirty quickly.

3. **Choose the phrase that most accurately describes the amount and distribution of your hair:**
   A. I have a lot of hair densely distributed over my scalp.
   B. I have a medium amount of hair evenly distributed over my scalp.
   C. I have a less-than-medium amount of hair sparsely distributed over my scalp.

4. **Individual strands of my hair are:**
   A. Large in diameter; my hair has volume and weight.
   B. Of medium size.
   C. Thin and fragile; my hair has little body and tends to be limp.

Answers to statements 1 and 2 generally match. If both answers are *A*, your hair type is dry; if both are *B*, your hair type is normal; and if both are *C*, your hair type is oily. Follow the instructions for your specific hair type throughout this section on hair care and styling.

If one of your answers is *B*, and the other is *A* or *C*, your hair is in the normal range, tending to either dryness or oiliness. Look for the instructions for your hair type tendency, either dry or oily, in the pages that follow.

If you answered *A* and *C* to statements 1 and 2, respectively, your hair condition ranges between the two extreme types, dry to oily. If you answered *C* and *A*, respectively, your hair ranges from oily to dry. These extremes may be caused by cleansing and conditioning products, hair coloring, or other chemical treatments. If you have either type of combination hair, you will probably want to follow the hair-care instructions beginning with the first word in your combination (although you should also consider the season and your lifestyle at the time you begin this care system). Take this inventory again in three months. If your hair falls more into the normal range at that time, adjust your hair care accordingly; if your hair has not improved noticeably, try the hair-care instructions beginning with the second word in your combination type.

If you use coloring agents or treat your hair chemically, take this inventory one week after treating it to note changes in your hair so you can adjust your hair-care routine.

If your answer to statement 3 was *A*, your hair distribution is thick and the quantity large; *B*, medium distribution and medium quantity; *C*, thin distribution and small quantity.

If your answer to statement 4 on hair texture was *A*, you have coarse hair; *B*, medium hair; *C*, fine hair.

The quantity and texture of your hair are not related to its type or condition. Although you can't radically change these characteristics, you can make your hair seem more — or less — full, softer, or coarser by following special hair-care guidelines and selecting appropriate hairstyles.

Record the characteristics of your hair in the spaces provided below. As you read the following pages on hair care and hair styling, refer to this inventory for these characteristics. Look for special considerations for your hair type, texture, distribution, and quantity; these qualities can influence your hair's strength, elasticity, and general appearance.

The hair of the woman at top is coarse in texture; below, the woman's hair is fine in texture.

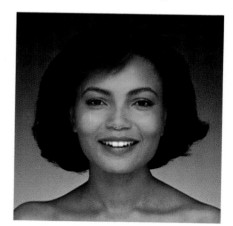

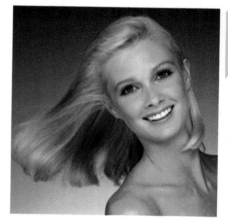

Hair type _____

Distribution/quantity _____

Texture _____

$\mathcal{D}$iscovering Your Hair Type

Your type of hair — dry, normal, or oily — is, like your type of skin, largely determined by heredity. In fact, most people have the same hair and skin types. If your skin is dry, your hair is apt to be dry as well; if you have oily skin, you probably have oily hair. But skin is also affected by the environment in which you live. The oil glands in the area below the scalp have the most influence on the condition of the hair strands themselves. This natural oil is secreted onto the hair shafts in the follicles, and both the amount and distribution of this oil are what determine the dryness or oiliness of your hair.

The water in the tissue below the scalp is responsible for supplying your hair and scalp with its healthful moisture content, which contributes mainly to the elasticity and, somewhat less, to the shine of your hair as well as to the condition of your scalp.

With consistent and proper care, you can make the most of your hair's unique characteristics — and even improve its condition. After taking the personal inventory of hair type on pages 146 and 147, you will be able to identify the special problem of your hair and care for it accordingly.

Dry hair is the result of insufficient oil and moisture in and around the hair shafts. This type of hair is often brittle and breaks easily. While dry hair may seem to grow more slowly, its constant breakage actually prevents it from growing very long. Also, because dry hair tends to fray at the ends, "split ends" can often result. Split ends occur when the cortex of the hair shaft cracks and splits into many tiny fibers. These filamentlike fibers at the shafts' ends catch among other split ends, causing tangling and further breakage when the hair is combed. Regular trimming of split ends should be combined with conditioning to help smooth the cuticles. Moisture and oil are retained on the hair shafts, making them silkier, more slippery, and less likely to tangle.

Bleaching, coloring, and permanent curling of the hair all tend to make it drier and, in some cases, more fragile. If your hair is chemically treated, check the special considerations on pages 154 to 159 to determine the specific care your hair requires.

Normal hair has a proper amount of oil and moisture on the scalp and in and around the hair shafts. Normal hair tends to have good elasticity and shine, with little or no breakage or split ends.

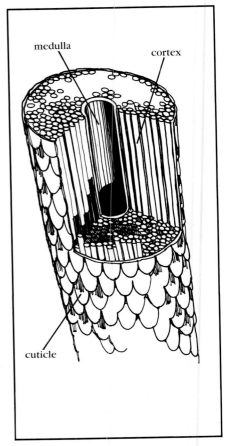

A shaft of your hair is composed of three layers. The cuticle or outer layer is made of hard transparent cells that overlap each other. The cortex or middle layer is composed of protein fibers and is protected by the cuticle. The medulla or center is a partially hollow structure. In some hair shafts, it is normal for the medulla to be absent or interrupted.

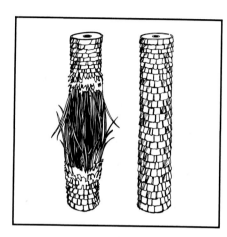

The shine of your hair is determined in part by the condition of the cuticle. When intact, the cuticle's scales form a smooth, even surface that reflects light. When damaged, the scales peel away from the hair shaft; light is not reflected and hair no longer appears shiny and lustrous. A split end — or a mid-shaft split, as shown at left — results from the unraveling of the ropelike fibers of the cortex when the cuticle is damaged.

Regularly cleansing the scalp and hair removes surface soils and helps keep your scalp operating well; moderate conditioning also helps your hair retain its important oil and moisture content. This moisture protects normal hair from the effects of dry environments, as well as from potentially damaging styling techniques such as blow-drying and permanent waving. In general, good hair care helps to maintain normal hair at its beautiful best.

Oily hair tends to be overly lubricated, limp, and lacking in shine as a result of excess oil production from the underlying sebaceous glands. Since both the scalp and the hair become somewhat sticky from the extra oil that coats them, soils stay on the surface of the scalp and hair shafts, contributing to the dull appearance of the hair. You must cleanse oily hair frequently and properly to remove these soils and give your hair added shine. Regular cleansing also helps to control the extra oils on the scalp and hair. Overly oily hair may not require much conditioning, but you may need to use a conditioner occasionally after shampooing to aid you in combing your wet and fragile hair.

Blow-dryers and electric curlers can dry the ends of hair shafts, which are less well supplied with the extra oils produced on the scalp. This results in what appears to be "combination" hair — oily scalp combined with hair that is dry at the ends. If you have combination hair, use conditioners only at the ends of your hair. A good program of hair care can also help normalize oil distribution.

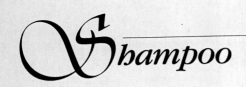hampoo

Keeping your hair clean is important to its appearance and to the health of your scalp. Cleansing removes perspiration, soil, and other impurities that stick to your scalp and interfere with its healthful functioning. Shampooing your hair also has obvious beauty benefits: clean hair smells fresh, feels wonderfully silken, and has a lustrous shine and healthy bounce. In order to cleanse your hair properly, you must use the right shampoo for your hair type and condition, and follow the proper procedure for shampooing.

The best shampoos have an acid to neutral-acid pH. Because the surface coating of oils and sweat has an acidic pH, these shampoos are compatible with your hair and leave it clean, soft, smooth, and shiny.

Dry to normal hair needs a gentle cleanser that removes soil without stripping away the oils and moisture that are vital.

Oily hair needs a more active cleanser because the shampoo must remove excess oil and soil from the scalp and hair strands.

How to Shampoo Your Hair Wet your hair and scalp thoroughly with warm water. Pour a small amount of shampoo — a dollop about the size of a quarter — into your palm, then rub your hands together to distribute the shampoo over your palms and fingertips. Don't pour shampoo directly from the bottle onto your hair because you will concentrate it on a single area. Apply the shampoo, working it into a lather with your fingertips. Gently massage your scalp with the balls of your fingers in a circular movement — never scrub with your nails; that could scratch and damage your scalp's delicate surface. Also, never pile your hair on top of your head; instead, allow shampoo and water to run down through your hair. Finish your shampoo by rinsing your hair and scalp thoroughly with clear, warm water, using your fingertips to separate strands of hair. Allow the water to run through your hair for at least thirty seconds to make sure all shampoo is rinsed away.

If your hair is oily, reapply shampoo if necessary following the procedure described above, then rinse again thoroughly for about thirty seconds. For a final rinse — and to harden your hair shafts — let cool water run over your hair and scalp for about ten seconds.

When your hair is thoroughly cleansed, you are ready to apply conditioner.

Keep in Mind . . .

Thick hair is dense and may tangle easily. Be sure to distribute shampoo gently and evenly, lifting hair up to apply shampoo underneath and on the scalp. Rinse very thoroughly, making sure to remove shampoo from scalp and hair.

Because clean hair appears to have greater volume, shampooing benefits *thin hair* by making it look thicker. Thin hair shafts are fragile, however, so shampoo should be applied very gently and distributed evenly, with as little manipulation of the scalp as possible.

Coarse hair tends to absorb shampoo readily and should be given an extra final rinse to remove all traces of suds.

Fine hair has more body when it's clean, so shampoo it often. Fine hair is very delicate, however, and breaks easily when it's wet. Shampoo gently, using light fingertip movements from scalp to ends.

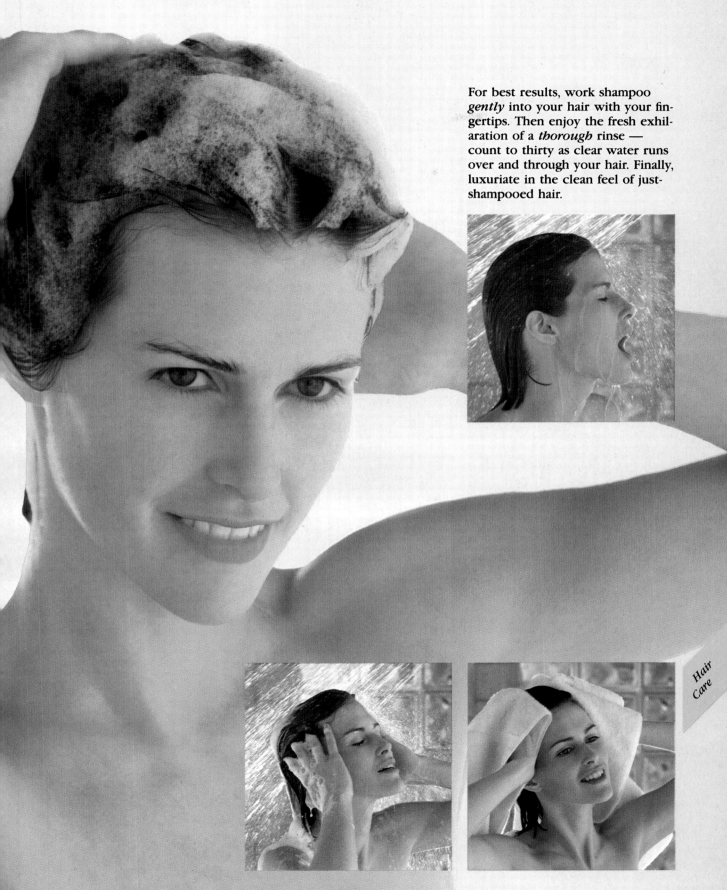

For best results, work shampoo *gently* into your hair with your fingertips. Then enjoy the fresh exhilaration of a *thorough* rinse — count to thirty as clear water runs over and through your hair. Finally, luxuriate in the clean feel of just-shampooed hair.

Hair Care

151

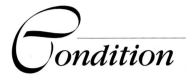

Condition

To keep hair shiny and flexible, all types have to be conditioned after shampooing. Natural oils from the scalp coat each strand of hair to give it shine and to seal moisture into the hair shaft. Moisture helps maintain elasticity and strength. Since dry hair does not produce enough natural oil to give the individual strands their protective and beautifying oil coat, a conditioner adds to the natural oil supply and gives dry hair shine as well as bounce and strength. Oily hair, however, may not have sufficient shine because too much oil coats the hair shafts, which are dulled by soil that sticks to them. Shampoos for oily hair remove some of the excess oil while removing soil; a conditioner restores the oil coating on the hair shafts to a normal level.

The best conditioners have an acid pH that is compatible with the scalp's natural acid level. A protein conditioner helps repair damage and strengthen the individual strands of hair. A good conditioner also minimizes tangling by helping smooth the outer layer of each hair shaft with a light coating. An acid pH protein conditioner can give extra body and fullness to oily hair. While protein conditioners are suitable for all types of hair, the method of application is different for each type.

How to Condition Your Hair After shampooing, gently squeeze out excess water from your hair. Pour about one tablespoon of conditioner into your palm and rub your hands together to distribute conditioner over your palms and fingertips. If you have ***dry to normal hair***, work the conditioner into your hair, beginning at the ends and distributing it evenly up over the shafts to the roots; if your ends are very dry and/or split, carefully massage extra conditioner into them with your fingertips. Leave the conditioner on your hair for at least one minute, then rinse your hair and scalp thoroughly and gently with clear, warm water for at least sixty seconds. Continue rinsing until all conditioner is removed and your hair feels smooth and slippery, but not greasy.

If you have ***oily hair***, begin at your hair ends and work the conditioner gently up the hair strands toward the roots, stopping midway between your hair ends and roots. Avoid getting conditioner on your scalp. Leave the conditioner on your hair for at least one

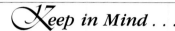

Keep in Mind . . .

Thick hair benefits from regular conditioning, which reduces its tendency to tangle when it is wet. Distribute conditioner evenly, lifting hair to make sure all of it receives conditioner.

Thin hair may be fragile and pull out easily, so distribute conditioner evenly without handling your hair excessively.

Conditioner helps ***coarse hair*** by adding extra shine and making it manageable. If your ends tend to fray and split, leave conditioner on ends one minute longer for added conditioning.

Conditioned ***fine hair*** has more body. Apply conditioner very gently in the direction in which your hair grows. Rinse thoroughly, since conditioner left on fine hair can add to its limpness.

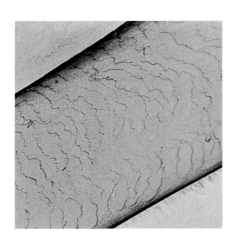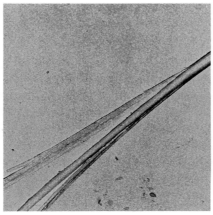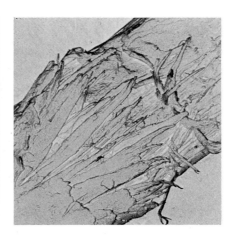

Conditioning adds bounce, softness, and luster to every type of hair. For problem hair, a conditioner is essential after every shampoo. Conditioning smooths the rough outer surface, or cuticle, of damaged strands, and prevents the tangling that can cause further breakage and damage. The photos above show, from left to right, a conditioned hair strand, a split end, and a mid-shaft split.

minute, then rinse thoroughly with warm (not hot) water. Continue rinsing until all conditioner is removed and your hair feels smooth and slippery, but not oily. A final cool-water rinse of your hair and scalp may provide some astringent action and help harden your hair shafts.

How to Dry Your Hair Hair strands are weakest when they are wet and can break or fray easily from hard rubbing with a towel. To prevent tangling and breakage, blot your hair gently with a soft, clean, fluffy towel, pressing gently against your scalp. Then smooth the towel along the length of your hair in the direction in which it grows. Circular or back-and-forth movements tangle your hair, resulting in breakage when you comb out wet hair.

Hair Care

Special Considerations

Regular conditioning after every shampoo can keep your hair healthy. But if your hair becomes seriously damaged, an intensive protein-packed conditioner instead of your regular conditioner can help restore shining flexibility.

Hair becomes dull and loses its bounce when the outer layer, or cuticle, of individual hair strands breaks. Intact, the cuticle's scales make a smooth, even surface that reflects light and gives hair a nice sheen. When the cuticle is damaged, the scales peel away from the hair shaft, preventing light from reflecting evenly and making hair look dull. Once the cuticle is damaged, moisture evaporates from the inner layer of the hair shafts and makes hair brittle, coarse, and dry. Whatever your hair type — dry, normal, or oily — the shafts and ends may become damaged and dry out for many reasons.

Hair can become seriously damaged by regular exposure to excessive sun and/or wind; by home or professional color treatments, including those that lighten or highlight; by permanent waving or curling, chemical relaxing or straightening; or by the use of electric appliances — blow-dryers, curling irons, rollers, hair dryers — several times a week. If you subject your hair to one or more of those appliances, or if your hair is very dry, you should use an intensive conditioner for your specific hair type.

Dry hair should receive an intensive conditioner once a week. After shampooing and lightly towel-drying your hair, apply intensive conditioner from the roots of your hair to the ends of the shafts. Place about one tablespoon of intensive conditioner in your hand, distribute it over your palms and fingertips, and apply it to your hair, working it gently into the strands and distributing it evenly. Leave it on for ten to fifteen minutes; rinse thoroughly.

Normal hair should receive an intensive conditioner twice a month. After shampooing and lightly towel-drying hair, apply intensive conditioner from the roots of your hair to the ends of the shafts, following the same procedure given for dry hair.

Oily hair should receive an intensive conditioner once a month. Apply intensive conditioner to the ends of your hair, working it up the hair shafts to midway between hair roots and ends. (Try not to get intensive conditioner on your scalp.) Leave it on for ten to fifteen minutes. Rinse thoroughly and follow with a cool-water rinse over your hair and scalp.

Keep in Mind . . .

If you wish to increase the manageability of *thick hair,* consider using an intensive conditioner instead of your regular conditioner after every other shampoo. Follow the recommended procedure for your hair type or condition.

Distribute intensive conditioner evenly through *thin hair* without excessively handling your hair or scalp.

Intensive conditioner adds shine and helps prevent *split ends.* Use intensive conditioner after every second shampoo, particularly on your hair ends, following the recommended procedure for your hair type or condition.

Intensive conditioner helps to strengthen and increase the elasticity of *fine hair.* Use intensive conditioner as directed for your hair type.

To protect your hair from the potentially damaging effects of blow-dryers, electric rollers, curling irons, and other appliances, use a protein-packed intensive conditioner regularly.

Combing and Brushing Your Hair

Along with environmental conditions and certain products and appliances, improper combing and brushing can damage your hair.

Comb — never brush — wet hair. (Brushing can snap wet hair shafts when they are most fragile.) Always use a wide-toothed comb with round, smooth teeth that won't snag your hair or scratch your scalp. Comb wet hair from the ends, working out knots and tangles at the bottom of the hair shafts. Lift up segments of hair to work out any tangles underneath. Never pull hard on tangled ends — you'll break individual hair shafts and you may actually pull hair out from its roots. When all the tangles are out, gently run the comb through your hair from the roots down to the ends.

After your hair dries, brushing is beneficial because it helps distribute the natural oils produced in the scalp onto the hair shafts. Brushing can be especially good for **dry to normal hair**, which may not be coated with sufficient oil to keep the hair strands smooth and elastic. If your hair is very **oily**, however, avoid brushing against your scalp. Rather, begin brushing your hair about an inch off your scalp to distribute the oil near your scalp on the ends of hair shafts.

If your hair is **thin**, avoid brushing your scalp. Your hair follicles may be fragile and hair shafts can be pulled out easily.

Fine hair is too delicate and easily broken to withstand much brushing. If your hair is very fine and you need to distribute more oil on your hair shafts, brush very gently and slowly, using a natural bristle brush with widely spaced bristles — or simply comb.

The best brush for all types of hair is one with natural, smooth-ended bristles in well-spaced rows. If your hair seems to catch or snag on the ends of bristles, your brush is probably worn and the bristles frayed or split. This usually means it's time for a new brush.

It's important to keep combs and brushes very clean. About once a week, soak plastic combs and brushes in a solution of one tablespoon of ammonia (or any strong household cleanser) to two quarts of warm water for an hour. For natural bristle brushes use a solution of diluted shampoo. The solutions loosen soil and remove stray hairs trapped on the surfaces of combs and brushes. Rinse combs and brushes thoroughly after soaking and dry them with a clean towel.

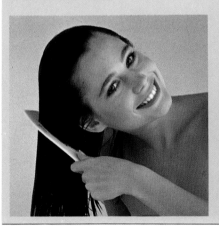

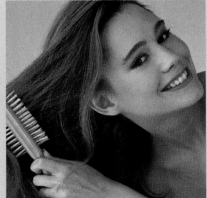

Special Considerations

No matter how well you care for your hair, you may discover problems that do not respond to your regular hair-care routine. Difficulties such as dandruff, dry scalp, and hair loss require special treatment. Because many hair and scalp problems may stem from your overall physical condition and be symptoms of a more serious disease, consult your doctor whenever you notice a serious or prolonged change.

Dandruff results in large, loose flakes that accumulate on the scalp and stick to the hair or fall to the shoulders. The disorder is caused by a problem with the reproduction rate of the scalp cells: they multiply much faster than they normally should and reach the surface before they are fully mature. Because the underdeveloped cells have not separated, they flake off in large clumps, rather than as tiny, barely noticeable flakes.

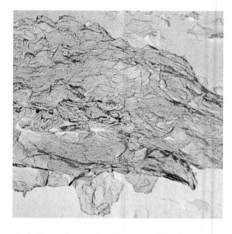

A flake of dandruff, magnified thousands of times.

There is no known preventive treatment for dandruff, and medical experts disagree as to whether the condition is associated with an overly oily or overly dry scalp. Some authorities believe there may be two different types of dandruff, one relating to dryness and one to oiliness.

Nor is there a known cure for dandruff, although there are ways to control it. Compounds such as zinc pyrithione and selenium sulfide, which help scalp cells reproduce at a normal rate, are available in several over-the-counter shampoo formulas. Active compounds such as salicylic acid are also among the ingredients of dandruff shampoos, which help break down and remove scalp cells as they come to the surface.

Dry scalp, as mentioned above, may or may not be a cause of dandruff. Similar to dry skin on any other part of the body, dry scalp may result in minor flaking, not unlike the flaking associated with dry facial skin. You can control dry scalp most effectively by using a very gentle shampoo and an intensive conditioner regularly.

Temporary hair loss can be a result of a number of factors. As new strands of hair form, they loosen and push dormant hair out of the follicles. So it is natural for some of your hair to fall from your scalp during shampooing or brushing. You normally lose about fifty to a hundred strands of hair each day. More than this amount of hair loss could result from any one of a number of factors and may be cause for concern.

Daily repetition of certain hairstyles — especially hair tightly pulled back, braided, or wrapped around rollers — can pull out individual hairs. Over time, such pulling can damage and destroy follicles completely; the hair will not grow back.

Emotional stress may bring on *alopecia areata,* a disorder that results in bald patches on the scalp and may be associated with changes in the immune system. Emotional stress can also cause hair to fall from all parts of the scalp.

Body stress — from high fever or lengthy surgery, for example — is also known to cause excessive hair loss, and evidence exists that medication for high blood pressure and psychological depression can cause hair to shed more rapidly than is normal. In addition, hair loss can result from pregnancy (it usually appears after delivery) or begin when a woman stops taking birth control pills. Hormonal changes that occur during pregnancy and while using birth control pills cause more hair follicles to remain dormant. After a woman gives birth, or when she discontinues using birth control pills, the renewal growth cycle begins, and the "old" hairs are pushed out and shed by the new growth. This cycle can continue for up to six months following pregnancy and delivery. Some women also notice that their hair becomes much drier during pregnancy. The condition is best controlled by using a very gentle shampoo and an intensive conditioner — instead of a regular conditioner — as often as after every other shampoo.

Most hair loss is temporary, but when the follicles are destroyed by serious scalp burns, excessive exposure to x-rays, or viral infection, hair loss can be permanent.

Special Considerations

The natural color of your hair is determined by the same pigments that determine the tone of your skin. As we grow older, the pigment-producing melanocyte cells may produce less, resulting in graying of the hair.

Your age at the time your hair begins to turn gray is largely a factor of heredity, as are all aspects of your natural hair color. When hair turns gray, it also may become dry, generally because the amount of oil produced in the scalp decreases as we get older. Increased use of an intensive conditioner can benefit dry hair, as can the use of a gentle shampoo for dry to normal hair.

Premature graying is an inherited characteristic; it may or may not be accompanied by dry hair. If your family history includes early graying, your hair could gray at almost any point in your life, sometimes as early as your late teens.

Gray hair can be very attractive, but if you prefer not to have gray hair or wish to change your hair color for any reason, many coloring options are available to you.

Chemical treatments for hair — including single- and double-process hair color, straightening or relaxing curly hair, and permanent waving — alter the structure of the inner layer of hair shafts. The chemicals lift up and penetrate the outer layer. As a result, hair may appear drier, more brittle, or less vital than before treatment because the scales that form this outer layer are damaged and do not reflect light evenly.

The physical effect of chemical treatments also causes individual strands of hair to increase in diameter and become more porous, especially at the ends. If your hair is thin and/or fine in texture, chemical treatments can add desirable body to your hair by expanding the shafts, making your hair look thicker and coarser. If your hair is very thin, fine, and fragile, however, strong chemical treatments may weaken it further, causing breakage. If you are not sure how fragile your hair is, ask a professional hairdresser how well the distribution and texture of your hair will react to chemical treatments.

Hair coloring agents such as henna, which coat your hair shafts without changing their outer layer, are another coloring option. Henna can deepen brown and black hair and add reddish highlights to all colors of hair. Henna tends to protect the hair's cuticle and

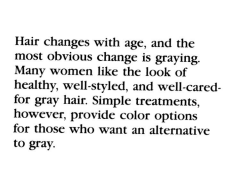

Hair changes with age, and the most obvious change is graying. Many women like the look of healthy, well-styled, and well-cared-for gray hair. Simple treatments, however, provide color options for those who want an alternative to gray.

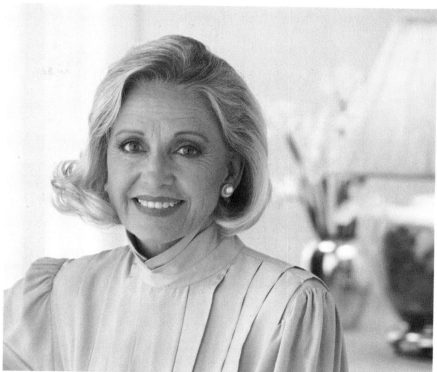

makes hair appear thicker and glossier. Neutral hennas add no color, but still make thin and/or fine hair appear to be thicker and have more body. Henna does not take well, however, on blond or gray or coarse hair, all of which absorb too much color and may be dulled by the henna colorants.

Conditioners applied immediately after chemical treatment help smooth the cuticle layer so hair becomes shinier and more flexible. Conditioners can help prevent hair that has been colored with a double-process method, or colored and permanent-waved, from breaking.

Some chemicals used in hair coloring, waving, or straightening formulas irritate the scalp. To prevent irritation or allergic reactions, professional beauticians often apply a protective cream to the scalp before applying the chemicals to the hair shafts themselves. If your scalp is sensitive, ask your hairdresser to use a cream before your chemical treatments.

Coloring and permanent waving products designed for at-home use are generally not as strong as those used by professionals. As a result, protecting your scalp may not be necessary, but it is still a good idea to keep the treatment on your hair and away from your scalp. Always test a patch to check for a possible allergic reaction.

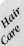

Hair Care

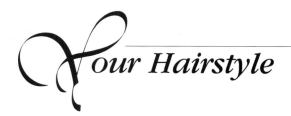

Your Hairstyle

On pages 160 to 163 we'll look at what role the shape of your face and various style elements play in choosing a hairstyle. But your lifestyle is a major determinant. If you wash, condition, and style your hair every morning, a short haircut may be best for you because it takes less time to care for. If you exercise three times a week or more, you may find short hair more manageable and easier to keep clean than long hair.

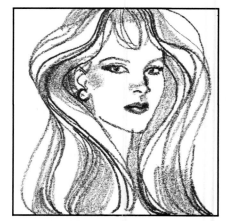

If you have plenty of time for hair care and find that your hair holds a flattering style for several days at a time, you may prefer to wear your hair long — pulled back from your face in a tidy knot for business days or styled in lavish curls for special nights out.

The distribution and quantity of your hair also play a part in your choice of hairstyle. Short or layered cuts make thick hair more manageable. A blunt cut adds thickness to thin hair, especially if you wear it medium length to your chin. Very short cuts and very long cuts can make thin hair look thinner, unless you add volume with curl.

The texture of your hair is another factor in selecting a style. Coarse hair often looks best short or, when worn long, thinned or layered. Because coarse hair holds curls and waves very well, it keeps a style longer than other types do and may not require too much styling time if you wear it long. Fine hair needs the body it gets from styles worn shoulder length or shorter. Longer styles tend to make fine hair look limp and shapeless, but permanent waves add both volume and body.

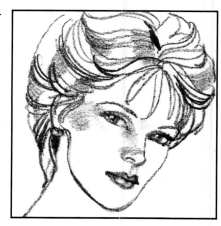

Longer hair is very versatile: you can wear it up for a sleek, sophisticated look or down for one that's full and feminine. Short hair is pert, pretty, and stylish; it's easy to care for and perfect for today's more active lifestyles.

The curliness or straightness of your hair should also be considered in your hairstyle choices. Very curly hair is easiest to manage when worn short. Wavy hair has a tendency to become curlier when it is short, and to become straighter as it grows. Straight and difficult-to-curl hair is best worn in simple styles — well-shaped short cuts, medium-length blunt cuts, or longer styles that can be pulled back, worn up in a knot or bun, or dressed up with accessories (see page 163).

Finally, your height should influence your choice of hairstyle. If you're tall, very short styles can make your face seem proportionately small; medium to longer lengths, worn full, offer better balance to a tall frame. If, in addition, you have a long neck, styles with greater length at the back are best. If you're short, long hairstyles tend to exaggerate your lack of height.

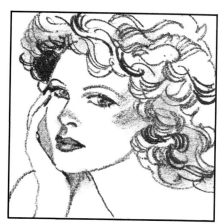

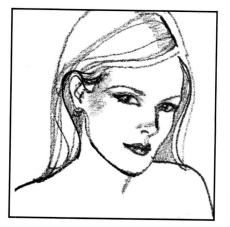

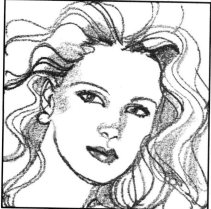

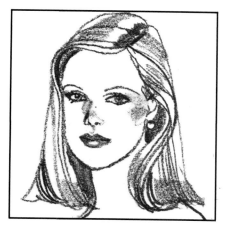

How you wear your hair — long, short, straight, curly, or wavy — will depend on your hair's natural characteristics and your own personal needs and preferences. The hairstyle that's right for you makes the most of your hair's best qualities.

Talking to Your Hairdresser

Here are tips on telling your hairdresser what look you want.

Think about what you want your hairstyle to do for you and explain it carefully to your hairdresser. Take along a picture of the style you want to try, but be sure it is appropriate for your hair type and face shape.

Listen to your hairdresser and have confidence in his or her opinions once you've found someone you like.

Speak up about the qualities of your hair. Does it hold curl well? Does it need extra body, shine, volume, a brighter color? Also, tell your stylist a little bit about yourself and your lifestyle: Do you have only ten minutes in the morning to style your hair? Can you handle a blow-dryer easily? Are your requirements different for work and play?

Be courteous. Book your appointments well in advance and, if you must cancel, give at least twenty-four hours' notice. And be punctual!

Be honest. If you don't like the work your hairdresser has done, tell the stylist why, as tactfully as you can. In many cases, the problem can be corrected before you leave the salon. And if you love what a hairdresser has done, tell that to him or her too! (A tip of 15 to 20 percent, except for a salon owner, also expresses your appreciation.)

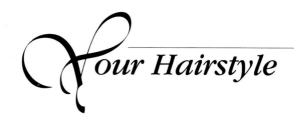

$\mathcal{Y}$*our Hairstyle*

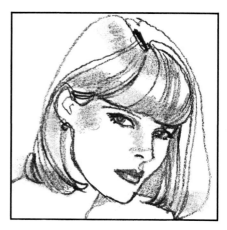 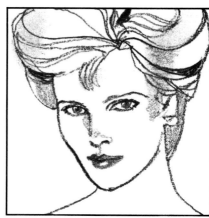

The way you wear your hair — parted, pulled back, with or without bangs — can affect the appearance of your features, highlighting and dramatizing them. Your personal style will always be a factor in the hairstyles you choose. Long styles and curls add softness and femininity. Short, straight hair has elegance and style. Hair worn back from your face and up off your neck is dressed-up and dramatic. Braids and ponytails are youthful and winsome. Very curly hair has a lively, spirited look. Wavy hair looks rich and distinctive.

Because hair-care technology offers so many options, you can make your hair look almost any way you want it to. Curly hair can be straightened and straight hair can be curled. Drab hair can be brightened, and unexciting hair colors can be lightened, darkened, or highlighted. Thin or fine hair can acquire more volume and body through special care and styling. Coarse or thick hair can be tamed and made softer and smoother by proper hair care and haircuts. Long hair can be cut shorter and short hair can be allowed to grow. What's most exciting about your hair is that there are so many possibilities to choose from.

To maximize the health and beauty of your hair, always start with a basic hair-care system designed for your hair type or condition. You can find one style you love and stay with it — or you can change your hair with the seasons, and experiment with color, length, style, curl, or wave. On the following pages, we show you how to put together all you've learned about hair care and style and make it yours.

Bangs worn straight across your forehead make your brow seem wider and draw attention to your eyes. Bangs that are long at the temples and curve up to a shorter length across your forehead also emphasize your eyes and make cheekbones look broader. Curly or wavy bangs soften angles on your upper face. The length of your bangs influences the appearance of your forehead: short bangs make the distance between eyebrows and hairline look longer than it is; long bangs make your forehead look shorter and sometimes wider.

Parts worn straight down the center add width to your brow, but may emphasize a long nose. Slightly off-center parts and side parts make your forehead seem narrower and can shorten the appearance of a long nose. Low side parts on your head broaden your forehead and help detract from your nose.

Hair pulled straight back or up off your neck draws attention to your facial shape. This style highlights your jawline, elongates and thins your neck, and can make your ears appear larger than they are. Drawing your hair over the tops of your ears when you wear it back from your face helps make your ears look smaller and closer to your head. Hair worn away from your face can also accentuate a small or large nose, an effect that can be diminished by wearing bangs across your forehead when you wear your hair back or up.

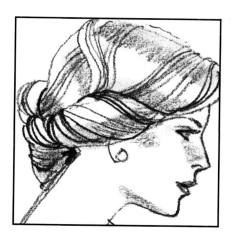

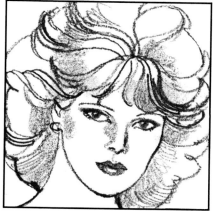

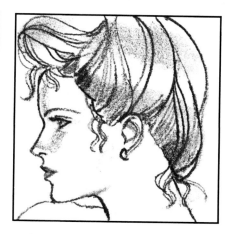

Fullness at the crown tends to make your face look longer; at your temples, fullness adds width to your cheeks and brow; and fullness at your jawline or below broadens your lower face. Waves or curls worn in styles that come in close on your face tend to make it look narrower; full hair brushed up and away from your face at your temples gives a lift to your cheekbones and makes your eyes look wider.

Tendrils — wisps of wavy or curly hair that fall from a pulled-up hairstyle — soften the outer edge of your face and add length to your neck. Tendrils can soften the severity of a hairstyle pulled back from your face.

Pretty Accessories for Your Hair

No matter what hair length or style you choose, accessories can add interest, color, and extra hold. **Barrettes** or **combs** capture stray hairs, hold hair away from your face, or flatten your hair. Or use combs to sweep hair up and back at your temples to give your whole face a lift. For easy height at your crown, push a comb upward at the top of your head. Select combs with round or softly pointed teeth and no sharp edges to snag or tangle hair. **Headbands,** and scarves or ribbons used as headbands, are great for taming hair that has

too much volume, or for holding hair when you're exercising. **Flowers** can be fastened in your hair almost anywhere. Cut the stems of fresh flowers to no more than two inches and secure them with bobby pins. If you like, glue a **ribbon** or **bow** onto a plain barrette, comb, or headband. Or tie ribbons around ponytails and braids to disguise covered elastics (plain rubber bands can break your hair).

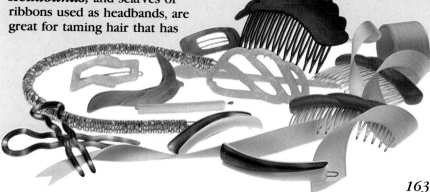

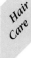

Taking a Closer Look

Use your hairstyle as a beauty accessory to complement those features of your face you wish to highlight, and to draw attention away from the features you wish to camouflage. Check the inventories on pages 92 to 95 to recall the aspects of your face you would like to enhance and those you are more interested in playing down. Then look for your basic facial shape in the drawings on these pages to find the most flattering hairstyle for you.

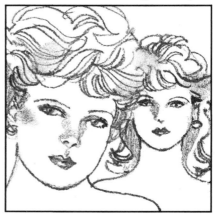 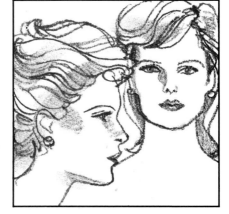

A ***round face*** benefits from a hairstyle that adds angles and helps conceal broad, round cheeks. Short hair should be at least as long as the bottoms of your earlobes, with most of your hair at the top and less on the sides, where your hair should be brought toward your face. Long hair should be worn with curls or waves surrounding your face, with most of your hair near your jaw, neck, or shoulders. Hair pulled straight back, worn in bangs, or cropped closely around the temples and cheeks accentuates roundness.

A ***square jaw and brow*** are best softened by a curly or wavy hairstyle that rounds off the angles of your face. Full, all-over curls should be at least as long as your jaw to detract from the squareness of your lower face. Off-center or swept-to-the-side bangs in soft curls or waves soften the wide angles of your brow. Curls or waves should be worn forward on the outer edges of your face from your forehead to your jawline to further soften your face. Straight hair worn in a blunt cut with straight bangs emphasizes hard-edged angles and can give your face an unbecoming geometrical flatness.

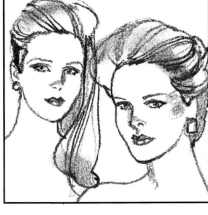 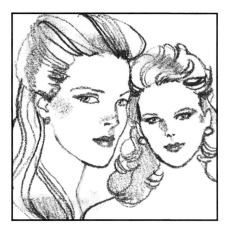 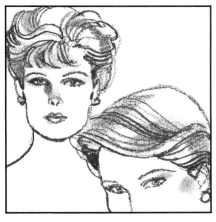

An **oval face** can be enhanced by a variety of simple hairstyles. Clean lines highlight this facial shape best; whether long or short, your hairstyle will be most flattering if you wear it straight or slightly wavy. Short styles look best worn away from your face, with most of your hair near your crown. Long hair is most flattering to an oval face when brushed or held back from your face. Or to break the regular lines of an oval face, wear your hair in a side ponytail at the nape of your neck or in an off-center knot near your crown. Few styles detract from the pleasant curves of an oval face, but hair worn very full at the sides can make your face appear too narrow and long. Hairstyles should be in proportion to the width of your face.

A **triangular face** can have a narrow jaw and wide cheeks and brow. The best hairstyles for this shape face are those worn close to your head, away from your face at your forehead and temples, with hair fuller from eye to chin level. If your hair is all one length, wear it pulled back at the top and softly waved or curled around your jawline. Or add weight and width to your lower face with a layered cut cropped short around your forehead and temples, and left full around your jaw, neck, and shoulders. Hair cut shorter than the bottoms of your earlobes and close to your face emphasizes wide cheeks and brow, diminishing a narrow jaw and small chin.

Another common **triangular face** has a broad jaw and narrow cheeks and brow. This face looks best with hairstyles worn full at your temples, with straight or waved bangs across the width of your forehead. A center or low side part also adds width to your brow. The best styles are short, at earlobe level or above, to bring the eye upward, away from your full jawline. Hairstyles that are straight or pulled back from your forehead and temples, and that fall at your jaw, exaggerate the greater width of your lower face and emphasize cheekbones that are too close together.

Putting It All Together

Karen has a part-time job that keeps her busy when she's not taking care of her home and family. She needs simplicity and ease from a hairstyle — her life is busy and she has to schedule hair care into a week that includes at least three exercise classes. For this reason, Karen keeps her style straight and simple and concentrates on regular trims every two months to control split ends and keep her cut well shaped.

Karen's hair type is normal, but it tends to get dirty easily because she exercises frequently. She finds her shower after each activity a good time to wash and condition her hair. She uses an intensive conditioner on the lower half of her hair strands twice a month after shampooing.

Karen has a medium quantity of hair that is very straight and difficult to curl. Her hair is also coarse to medium in texture and doesn't take permanents and sets evenly. For Karen, a blunt cut, at chin level, offers shape and style without requiring waves and curl. It also makes her hair look fuller and thicker than it actually is.

When she exercises, Karen ties her hair back in a ponytail and uses a headband under her bangs. For elegant evenings, she pulls back her hair in a braided twist at the nape of her neck, holding the sides with barrettes or fastening a flower next to the twist. Sometimes, for important days at work, she adds an off-center topknot, fastening the short stray ends at the sides and back with decorative combs.

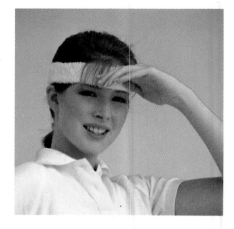

Karen's hair care and styling center around her lifestyle and the characteristics of her hair. With straight, hard-to-curl, somewhat coarse hair, she relies on an excellent haircut to give her the shape and style she needs. She uses an intensive conditioner and has her hair trimmed regularly to help her split ends problem. The length of her hair allows her to pull it up and off her face during strenuous activity, as well as dress up her hairstyle for special occasions. Good basic hair care keeps Karen's hair shiny, manageable, and soft; simple styling accentuates the natural qualities of her hair.

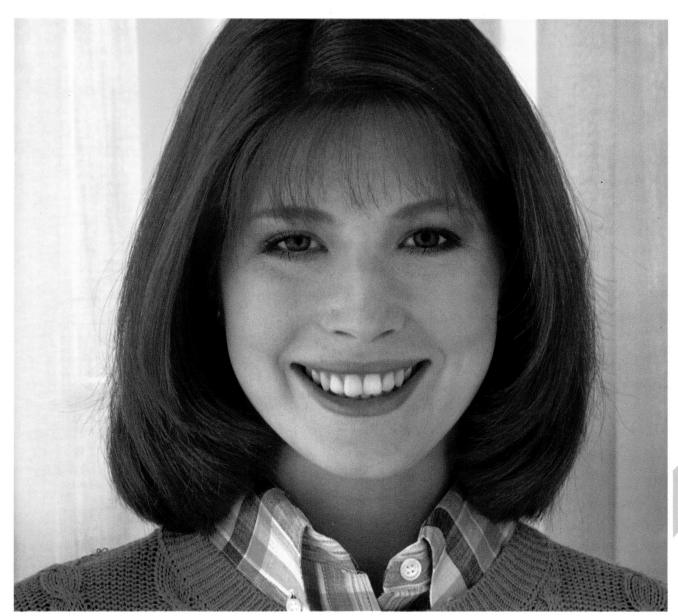

Putting It All Together

Janice needs a feminine and stylish look for her job and prefers the versatility of a long hairstyle. Her lifestyle also allows her enough time in the evenings to care for her shoulder-length blond hair.

Janice's hair is in the normal to dry range and doesn't need daily washing and conditioning. Because of its length, her hair requires time for proper washing and conditioning, so she sets aside two or three evenings a week for this purpose. She uses regular conditioner on her hair after every shampoo and applies an intensive conditioner after every third or fourth shampoo.

Her thick hair demands little special care. She finds that nightly brushing adds shine and helps distribute the oils from her scalp on the hair shafts. She takes extra care in combing her hair when it's wet because it tends to tangle easily.

Janice's medium-textured hair holds styles well because it's thick. Her hairdresser brightens its color with professional highlighting about once every three months, giving her hair a subtle lift of color. The highlighter makes her hair appear dry, so she makes sure she uses an intensive conditioner regularly.

Janice gets regular trims about four times a year (when she has her hair highlighted), and finds that her hair holds its shape nicely when she allows it to dry naturally. For casual weekends, she doesn't have to style it at all. But for the polished look she needs for her career, Janice uses a curling iron on mornings, after she's shampooed and conditioned, to add a fashionable upswept look to her style. After her hair is dry she sometimes lifts the side segments of hair to curl them up and back with the curling iron. Since her hair holds curl well, she only has to touch up the style occasionally between shampoos.

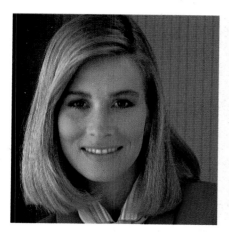

Janice helps maintain her strong, healthy hair with a basic hair-care system, taking the time to use an intensive conditioner regularly to counteract the drying effects the curling iron and the highlighting color treatments have on her hair. For casual days, she may braid her hair and tie the ends with pretty ribbons; for elegant evenings, she often wears her hair down and pulled behind her ears, giving her a youthful but stylish look.

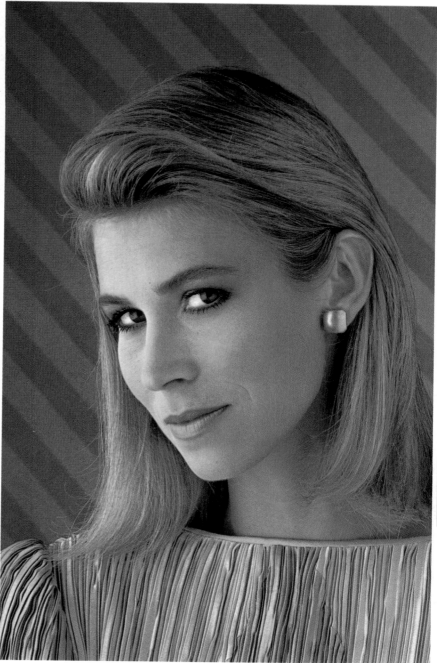

Hair Care

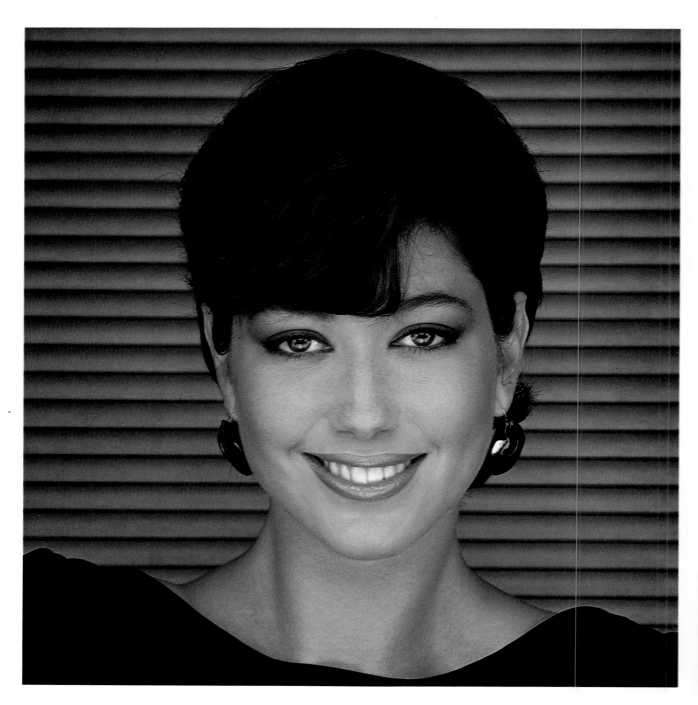

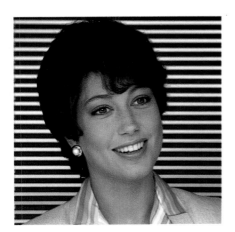

Daily shampooing and proper home and professional care keep Maryanne's hair shiny and soft. A good hair stylist gives Maryanne the style, shape, and color she wants, and the right hair-care system helps maintain her hair's healthy vitality and bounce.

Maryanne is a successful working mother who doesn't have much time for hair styling before she goes off to work. She wants her hair to look great all the time with as little care as possible.

Maryanne's oily hair needs frequent washing. Since it looks best right after shampooing, she finds it easiest and most beneficial to wash her hair every morning in the shower.

Because her hair is thin and she needs an easy-to-care-for style that will work for her every day, Maryanne keeps her hair short and permed. She conditions it daily to give her hair extra body and shine; once a month, she uses an intensive conditioner on the ends, which dry out from the permanent.

Maryanne consulted her hairdresser about ways to increase the body of her hair and improve its color. Because she usually gives herself home permanents for curl, and the chemicals can affect the hair color, she wanted a professional opinion on adding color. Her stylist didn't want to use a strong peroxide-based coloring agent on Maryanne's permed hair, so he suggested a deep auburn henna. The henna brightens Maryanne's natural coloring, while adding shine, body, and pretty highlights to her hair. She has her hair colored about every eight weeks, when she has it trimmed.

Maryanne finds she can style her hair quickly after her morning shampoo and conditioning. She carefully dries and combs through her hair, then fluffs it up with her fingertips. By the time she's put on her makeup, made breakfast for the baby, and dressed for work, her hair is dry and she's ready to leave for the office. For dressy occasions, Maryanne adds a flower-adorned barrette over one ear.

Hair Care

Body Care

Smooth, glowing body skin reflects the care and attention you give your body. By giving top priority to your health and well-being; getting enough sleep and exercise; taking time to relax; and finally, expressing your mood and personality through clothing and fragrance to create your unique sense of style, you show your concern for making your body its beautiful best.

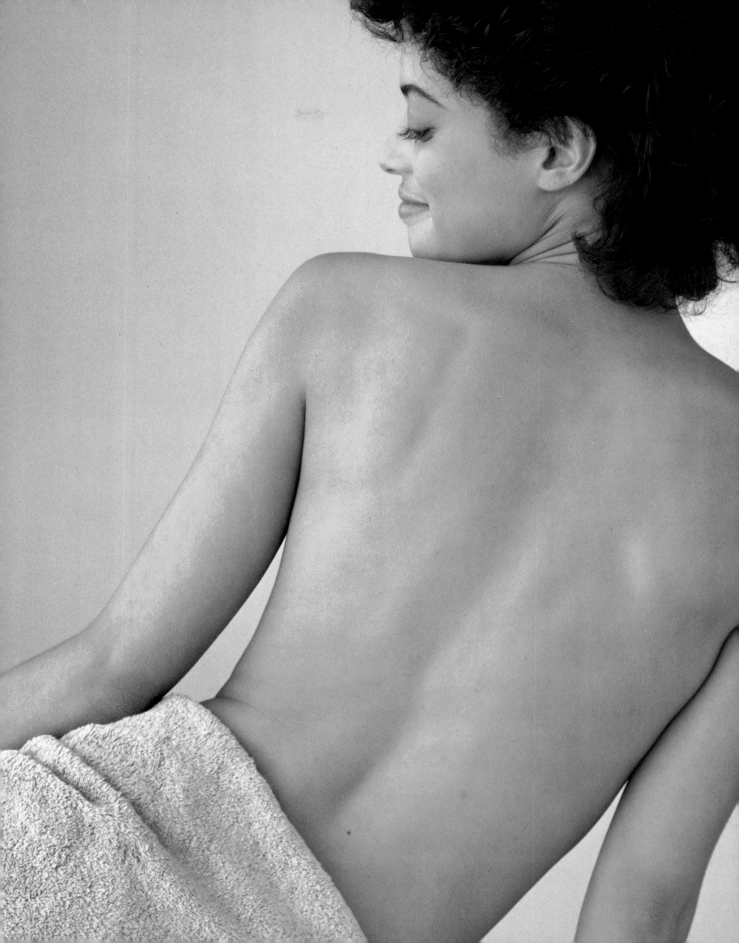

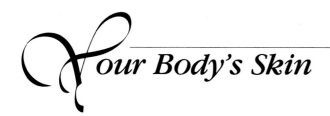our Body's Skin

The skin on your body is similar to that on your face in basic structure. But greater and lesser distribution of glands and tissues all over your body makes body skin function differently. You can clearly observe that the skin on your eyelids is quite different from the skin on the palms of your hands or the skin on your shoulders. Texture, hair growth, the presence of sebaceous (oil) and sweat glands, nerve endings, and amounts of fat and muscle vary widely over your entire body.

A good example of this variance is the distribution of oil glands that lubricate the surface of the skin. They are most prevalent in the skin of the face, scalp, and upper trunk, while no equivalent glands exist in the palms of hands or soles of feet. Similarly, sweat glands called the apocrine glands are almost exclusive to the underarms and genitals. These glands secrete a milky substance that, when broken down by bacteria on the skin's surface, produces the characteristic odor of human perspiration. The more common sweat glands, the eccrine glands, are far more numerous on the body. The palms of the hands, soles of the feet, and armpits contain the greatest number of eccrine glands; the head, trunk, and limbs have the next highest concentration.

The hands and feet are unique in that they produce fingernails and toenails, which are made of keratin, the same protein found in the epidermis and hair. In nails, keratin forms a thick, translucent plate, strengthening and protecting fingers and toes. The pale half-moon at the bottom of each nail is the root where cells push upward to form the hard nail. The cuticle — the small, somewhat tough fold of skin at the bottom of the nail — protects the area where new cells grow. Nails grow about one-tenth of one millimeter each day, and it takes six months for a nail to replace itself.

Some parts of the body are more sensitive to touch than others because of the kinds and distribution of nerve cells in the lower layers of body skin. Nerve fibers vary in thickness and sensitivity; thin nerve fibers may transport signals, or impulses, more slowly to the nervous system and the brain than do thick ones. In addition, when nerve receptors are close together — as on the fingertips and lips — they are more sensitive. When these fibers are farther apart — as on the backs of the hands — the skin may be less responsive to touch.

Skin, your largest organ, functions differently in various areas of your body. The skin covering your fingertips and lips, for example, is highly sensitive to touch; the soles of your feet contain a large concentration of sweat glands; the perspiration secreted by your underarms is different from that of most other parts of your body. The distinct nature of your body skin requires a beauty-care routine suited to its specific characteristics, functions, and needs.

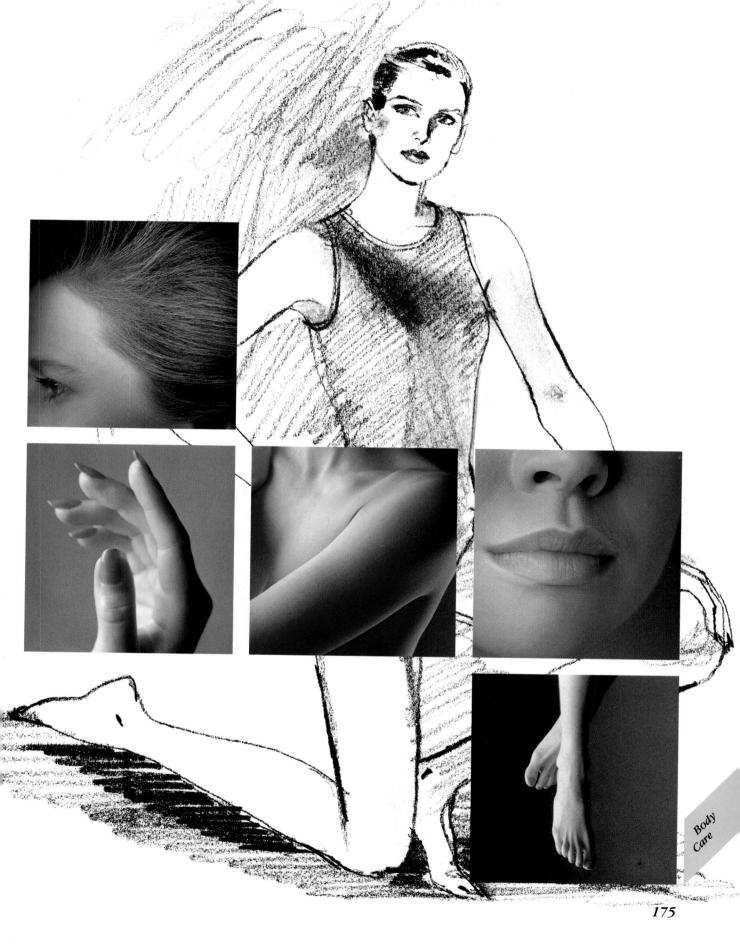

Body
Care

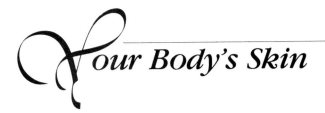our Body's Skin

Both facial and body skin are highly vulnerable to the damaging effects of the sun and need protection from ultraviolet radiation (see pages 68 and 69 and 190 and 191). The drying effects of the sun can be particularly harmful to your entire torso and arms and legs because this skin contains fewer sebaceous glands.

The skin on your body needs as much careful health and beauty attention as does the skin on your face. But because your body skin functions differently from your facial skin, your body skin-care routine needs to vary from the regimen for your face. For more specific differences between body and facial skin, refer to the chart on the opposite page.

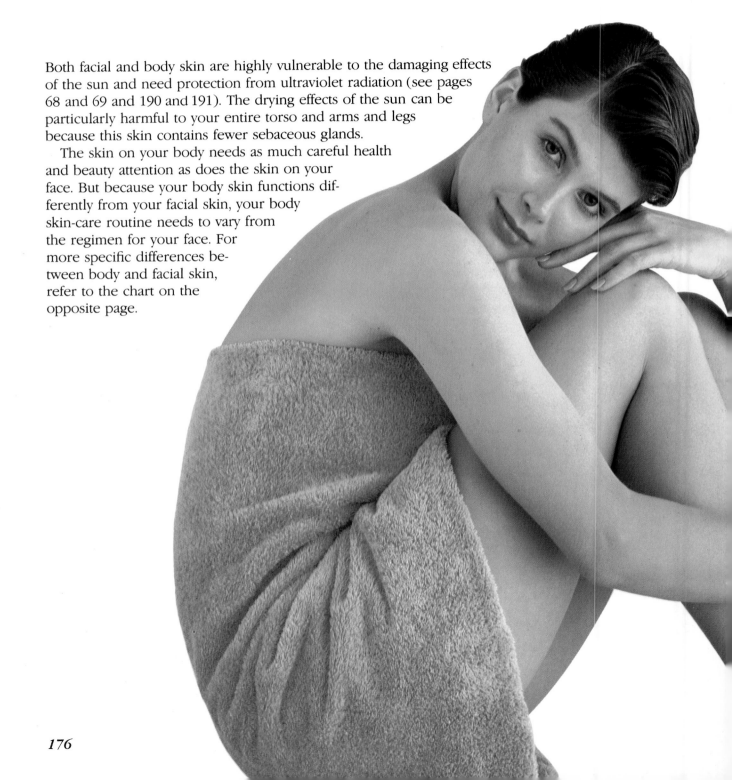

Your Skin from Head to Toe

Factors	Facial Skin	Body Skin
Aging	Your face is constantly exposed to the environment, including the sun and other factors that increase its potential for rapid aging.	You generally cover and protect your body skin with clothing, reducing the drying effects of the environment.
Oiliness	Many large sebaceous glands in the dermis provide skin with more surface oils.	Fewer and smaller sebaceous glands in the dermal layer tend to make skin dry.
Fat	The fatty layer and the dermis are thin, providing less protection from temperature changes and physical trauma.	The fatty layer is thick, in general, and may be very dense in certain areas of the body. Combined with a generally thick dermis, this adds greater support and insulation to surface skin.
Wrinkles	Muscles attached to skin layers are directly involved with the skin's movement. The frequent use of these many small muscles eventually results in lines forming on the surface skin. Also, more sun exposure means more wrinkles.	Muscles attached to underlying joints and bones may be quite large. Since large areas of the body move together, wrinkling tends to be minimal. Also, less sun exposure means fewer wrinkles.
Sensitivity	Nerve endings are close together, so receptivity to stimulation is greater.	Nerve endings are farther apart (except in the fingertips), resulting in reduced sensitivity to outside stimuli.

Body Care

177

Special Considerations

The skin that covers your body is a highly efficient organ that, with proper care, will stay healthy. Nonetheless, some conditions of body skin will not respond to even the most careful skin-care routine, and often require medical care.

Psoriasis can appear on any part of the body, although it most often develops on the scalp, knees, and elbows. It is characterized by patches, called plaques, of scaly, shedding skin that vary in size and range in color from red to white to silvery. Normal skin cells harden and die off when they reach the outer layer of the skin's surface. In psoriasis, however, the production of new cells below is too swift, and the surface skin begins to shed cells that are not completely hard and dead to make room for the new cells. It is estimated that psoriasis affects 2 percent of the American population. The condition is not contagious and, while it cannot be cured, it can be controlled in most instances through medical treatment by a dermatologist.

Eczema, medically known as *atopic dermatitis,* can cover a wide range of skin problems that are usually related to an extreme susceptibility to some form of irritation or are caused by an allergic reaction. Skin affected by eczema becomes dry, scaly, red, and very itchy, most often where the skin is sensitive, as on the insides of elbows and backs of knees. Eczema is believed to be hereditary and may be associated with other disorders, such as asthma, hay fever, and conjunctivitis. The eczema victim may also have a number of allergies and be supersensitive to soaps and detergents.

Prickly heat is known medically as *miliaria.* One form, *miliaria rubra,* results when underlying sweat glands become blocked, usually after prolonged exposure to hot, humid conditions. It is aggravated by the pressure of tight or binding clothing at the waist, shoulders, buttocks, and thighs, which does not allow perspiration to evaporate readily. Affected areas become red, irritated, and extremely itchy, sometimes producing a rash of small red dots. Prickly heat can usually be relieved by seeking a cooler, drier environment and wearing clothing that does not press against the skin.

Scarring results in a visible patch of new skin, different from the surrounding skin, and usually occurs over a large or deep area that has been cut. Because the skin is constantly regenerating new cells, superficial cuts and abrasions are usually repaired rather quickly. In

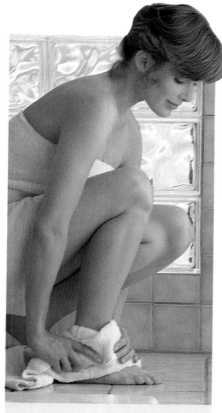

*A*thlete's Foot

Healthy human skin is populated with microorganisms that are usually harmless. However, the fungi that cause athlete's foot tend to multiply and cause an itchy, irritated rash between the toes and in the small crevices of the feet. While this fungus is always present on the skin, it can multiply rapidly in damp areas of skin. The result is the uncomfortable condition called athlete's foot, which is very contagious. The best precaution is to keep your feet clean and dry, particularly after they have been on surfaces where the fungi may have been deposited by others (locker rooms, showers). Over-the-counter topical ointments and powders can help clear up athlete's foot, but in severe cases, a physician should be consulted.

large and deep cuts, however, blood rushes to fill the cut area. This blood hardens into a clot that attaches itself to the sides of the cut and protects the new connective tissue and epidermis being produced from the surrounding skin. This tissue grows below the clot, filling in the space that remains while the clot shrinks.

Getting immediate medical attention for large cuts in the skin is the best way to prevent scarring. Treatments can close the cut skin and reduce the size of a scar. Once scars have formed, the most effective way to conceal them is cosmetically, by use of an opaque, masking foundation product. Scars that cover a large area on a highly visible part of the body and whose appearance is very disturbing may be improved through surgical techniques.

First-degree **burns** are the least serious, primarily affecting the upper layers of skin and resulting in redness from dilated blood vessels near the skin's surface. Second-degree burns produce blistering and the accumulation of fluid between the dermis and epidermis. In third-degree burns, both the epidermal and part of the dermal layers of skin in the affected area are destroyed, leaving the underlying tissue vulnerable to infection. Such burns are treated, in most cases, by skin grafting, a surgical process in which skin from another part of the body is moved to cover the area that has lost its skin. The transplanted skin adapts to the new area and grows out from its edges to form a new covering. The site from which the skin patch was taken simply regenerates skin cells to provide a new skin surface.

Body Care

Taking a Closer Look

Your body is affected by the way you live — how much exercise and sleep you get, how well you eat, how healthy you are, and how much attention you pay to yourself, like caring for your skin, hands, and feet. Just as your skin, makeup, and hair project the message that you feel good about yourself, so does the way you take care of your body. You'll want to do everything you can to keep your body toned and fit. The following inventory will guide you in evaluating your needs and goals.

1. **My usual day is:**
   A. Very active; I'm out and about, on my feet, and moving a lot.
   B. Mostly sedentary; I sit at a desk or other work station all day.
   C. A combination of active and sedentary.

2. **I usually have the most leisure time:**
   A. In the morning.
   B. At midday or in the afternoon.
   C. In the evening.
   D. On weekends.

3. **My favorite kind of exercise is:**
   A. Competitive sports (one on one or team games).
   B. Noncompetitive sports where I can improve at my own pace.
   C. Walking or other less strenuous activities.

4. **I sleep well at night and get plenty of rest:**
   A. Usually.
   B. Sometimes.
   C. Seldom.

5. **The area where I live is:**
   A. Urban.
   B. Suburban.
   C. Rural.

6. **The climate in my area (check all that apply):**
   A. Changes with the seasons in temperature and humidity.
   B. Is mostly humid.
   C. Is mostly dry.
   D. Remains quite cold.
   E. Remains hot and sunny.

7. **I would like to improve the way I take care of my:**
   A. Body skin.
   B. Hands and feet.
   C. Figure.

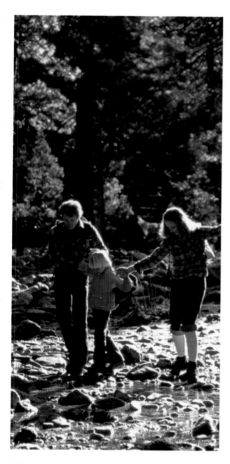

There are many forms of relaxation and exercise, and it is important to make time for all of them. Outdoor activities are necessary for your overall beauty and health.

Statement 1: Because fitness is one of today's beauty essentials, it's important to include some activity in your daily schedule. Where, when, how, and with whom you exercise depends on your personal preferences and needs; the key is making the commitment to stick with the regular program. If you work in an office, it's especially important to make exercise a priority in your day. Still, no matter what kind of work you do, you'll most likely find that exercise is an excellent way to refresh, relax, and unwind.

Statements 2 and 3: For optimum results, tailor your shape-up to fit your lifestyle. Determine what time is best for you — morning, midday, or evening — and select an appropriate activity. Whether you choose an early jog, a brisk lunchtime walk, or an evening tennis match, you'll want to plan ahead. Look closely at your schedule and know your limitations. If you need more discipline, sign up for a class or pre-book court time. Exercise with a friend or join group activities. Whatever you choose, make it something you enjoy. If you look forward to your exercise time — if you equate fitness with fun — the more likely it is your efforts will be successful.

Statement 4: Along with regular exercise, getting enough sleep is important to looking and feeling your best. The information on pages 204 and 205 addresses the need for proper sleep and relaxation. What you want to remember is that when you feel good —

when you've gotten enough sleep, you've taken time to relax, and you've included exercise in your day — you'll be more productive in everything you do.

Statements 5, 6, and 7: Along with staying fit, you want to keep your body skin in tiptop shape. No matter where you live — in the city, the suburbs, or the country — you need to protect your skin from the harmful effects of the sun. Included in the body-care section are tips for giving your body the protection it needs. Another big consideration is the climate you live in; pages 66 and 67 explain how to care for and protect your skin in all types of weather.

A beautiful body — fit, trim, smooth, soft, and well groomed — is an attainable goal. Make it yours with the direction, motivation, and effort offered on the following pages.

$\mathcal{B}$ody Skin Care

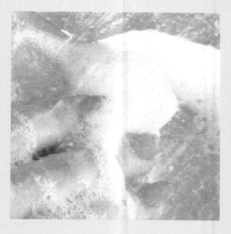

For body skin that glows with healthy radiance, you need to follow an effective, ongoing skin-care routine. Because its structure is different from that of facial skin, and because much of it is less exposed to the environment, body skin has somewhat different needs. Total body care begins with a basic four-step program that leaves you feeling wonderfully rejuvenated all over: softly polished shoulders, sleek, smooth arms and legs, beautiful hands, and pretty feet.

This scientifically based and uniquely balanced program to care for and beautify your body skin is based on these four simple steps: cleanse, buff, moisturize, and protect. When followed regularly, these steps will give you the beautiful body skin you want — clean, silky smooth, and glowing. Your body-care routine should feel refreshing, help your skin perform at its best, and leave your skin looking radiant and healthy.

Cleanse
Begin by gently washing away the daily buildup of surface dirt, oils, and impurities on your skin, using a rich gel that gently foams away soils while helping to soften the skin and maintain its natural acid balance. Proper cleansing should leave your skin feeling fresh and clean, not tight and dry.

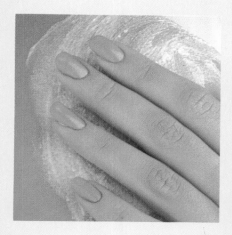

Buff ▲

After cleansing gently, use a buffing cream with a mild abrasive to whisk away dead surface cells, smooth rough calluses on heels, knees, hands, and elbows, and give a smooth, polished finish to your shoulders, arms, and legs. Like a facial mask for your body, buffing stimulates, smooths, and softens.

Moisturize ▶

After you have cleansed and buffed, apply a rich, creamy moisturizer to your shoulders, arms, torso, hips, buttocks, and legs — everywhere. Moisturizer helps lock in surface moisture, leaving skin soft and silky. It should not leave a greasy after-feel.

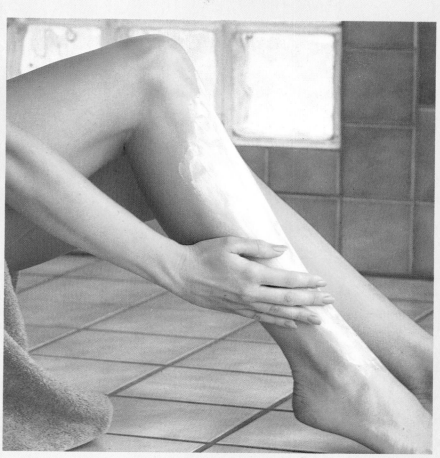

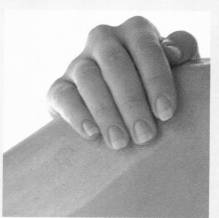

Protect

Beautifully cleansed, buffed, and moisturized skin needs protection from the sun to maintain its youthful softness and glow. A sunscreening lotion with a sun protection factor of at least 10 guards your body skin against harmful ultraviolet rays and helps prevent the premature aging and dehydration caused by exposure to the sun.

Body Care

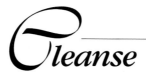

Cleanse

A regular cleansing routine is important to the overall health and glow of your skin. Perspiration from your body's sweat glands can be broken down by the normal bacteria present on your skin's surface to produce an unpleasant odor. Regular cleansing prevents perspiration and bacteria from accumulating.

Cleansing must be effective enough to get your skin really clean and, at the same time, gentle enough to help your skin retain its natural lubrication. A body cleansing gel gently foams away surface soils, perspiration, and bacteria without irritating or drying the surface of the skin. The rich foam also feels wonderful and rinses off easily, leaving the skin clean, silky, and refreshed.

How and When to Cleanse In the shower or bath, squeeze body cleansing gel on your wet hands and lather your entire body until you have worked up a rich foam. To help stimulate your skin and loosen dead surface cells, apply the gel to a body brush, natural bath sponge, or washcloth and gently scrub your body. (If your back is acne-prone or tends to break out, do not use an abrasive on it as this may further irritate the condition. A soft sponge is best for any area of the body that is easily irritated.)

As you cleanse, pay special attention to areas that have the greatest number of sweat glands and therefore tend to produce odors — the underarms, groin, and feet. When you use cleansing gel in your bath, pour it under the running water, as you would bubble bath, to get lots of rich suds. Lather your body well with the suds and put a bit more gel on your applicator to work up extra foam all over. Be sure to rinse well to remove all traces of lather. For a final rinse, take a quick shower.

What time of day you bathe is a matter of personal preference, but bear in mind that your body's sweat glands are active throughout the day, even in cold weather, because perspiration is activated by emotions as well as by the temperature. Cleansing is the first vital step in total body care. Keeping your skin clean makes it look attractive and function beautifully. The soft, silky feeling and fresh, light scent of just-washed skin will give you extra confidence all day long. Proper cleansing is the basis of your body skin care — the groundwork for the next important steps to follow.

Cleansing, your first step in body care, can be as good for your spirits as it is for your skin. Morning showers wake you up and help you start your day refreshed. Evening showers revitalize your spirits and help you go from day to evening. A bath before bed is relaxing and soothing, allowing you to slip between the sheets feeling wonderfully clean. In the bath or shower, a gently foaming body cleansing gel makes your skin feel baby soft, smooth and silky, and totally clean.

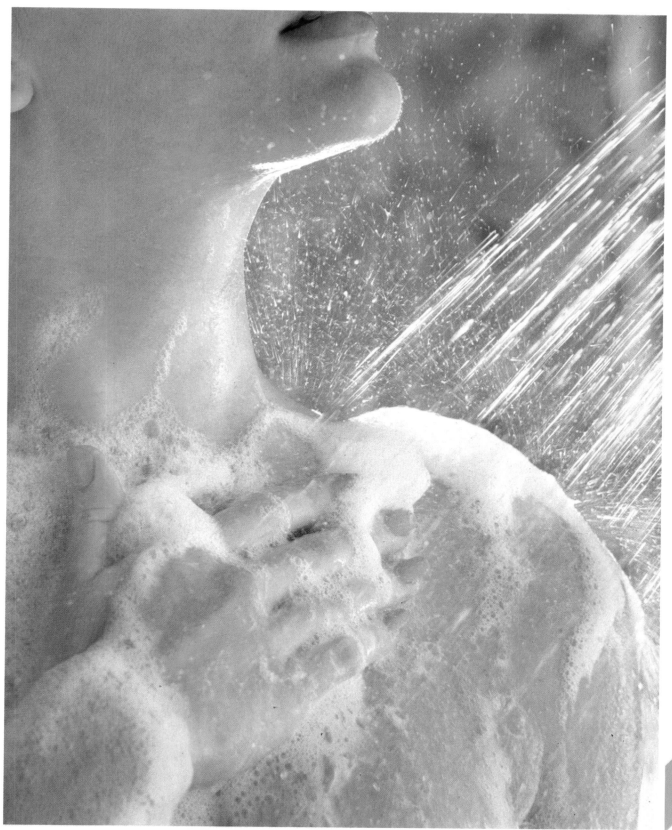

185

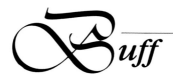

Buff

Your body skin, like your facial skin, is constantly renewing itself. As new skin cells are produced and move upward to form the top layer of the skin, they harden and die off to form the protective surface of the skin. Older cells separate from the skin's surface in tiny flakes or build up as a callus. To keep your skin clear and glowing and functioning properly, calluses should be removed.

Buffing body skin aids its natural cell-sloughing process (which tends to slow down with age) and leaves a fresh skin surface. Buffing also helps remove hard patches or calluses that form on elbows, knees, hands, or feet. Because the newly exposed skin must also be guarded against excessive loss of moisture, your buffing product should have a mild cream base. Extra-fine buffing grains in a rich formula help remove the dead cells that can dull the skin's natural glow. Buffing cream leaves your skin brighter, more translucent, and satiny to the touch.

How and When to Buff It's best to use buffing cream twice a week, or about every three days, immediately after washing with cleansing gel. Apply the cream to your fingers and spread it on your wet skin, concentrating on any calluses on your feet, elbows, or knees. Use the cream to smooth and polish your shoulders, arms, thighs, hips, and torso. Rub the buffing cream gently in a rotating motion, using your hands or a washcloth. Avoid irritated areas, skin that has broken out, and very thin or fragile skin — the underarms, breasts, groin, and inner thighs. Then, using light massaging movements with your hands or washcloth, rinse away all traces of buffing cream. If you have especially stubborn calluses or hard skin on your feet, elbows, hands, or knees, use the cream regularly on these particular areas.

Buffing is the second important step in your total body skin-care routine. Faithful use of a buffing cream will help your skin function healthfully and look and feel extra clean, soft, and lustrous.

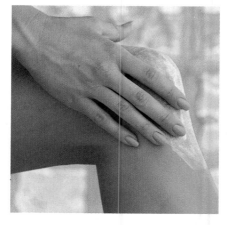

Like polishing your skin, buffing with a cream shines your shoulders, gives legs and hips a silken luster, and softens calluses on heels and elbows. And as it invigorates, it sloughs off dull surface cells. Buffed skin looks clearer, softer, and smoother and makes you feel wonderful about the special care you're giving your body.

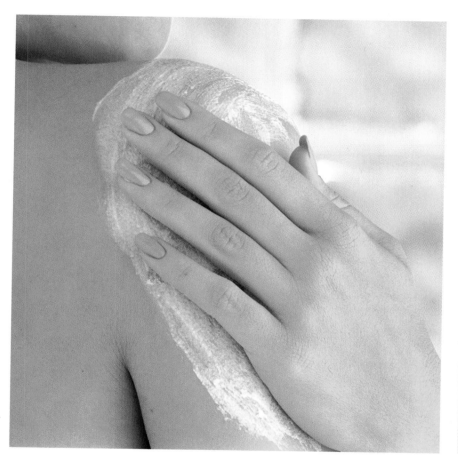

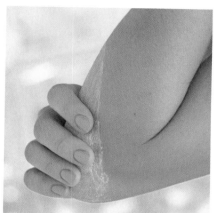

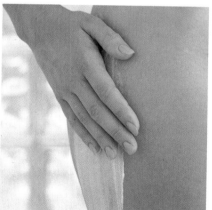

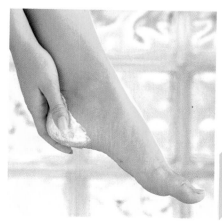

Moisturize

A square inch of your body skin has fewer oil glands than an area of facial skin the same size, so it may dry out easily no matter what your skin type. Body skin is also subject to much abuse. Tight or binding clothing can rub and irritate your skin. Shaving legs and underarms (see pages 198 and 199), because it allows moisture to evaporate from the skin, can contribute to dryness. To substitute for lost natural oils on your body skin, you should regularly apply a rich, creamy moisturizing lotion that disappears completely. A moisturizer should make your skin smooth and supple, with no greasy after-feel, and leave a fresh scent that won't interfere with other fragrances.

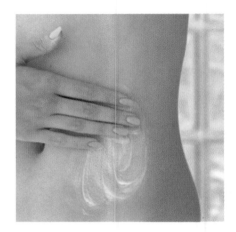

How and When to Moisturize After your shower or bath, gently towel dry your body, leaving it slightly damp. Pour a generous amount of body moisturizer into your hand and smooth it all over. When applied to damp skin, body moisturizer helps hold some water on the skin's surface. Massage the lotion gently onto your skin, covering your shoulders, chest, arms, waist, stomach, hips, buttocks, and legs. Pay special attention to drier areas, such as your lower arms, lower legs, feet, elbows, and knees. Continue spreading the lotion evenly all over until it disappears completely.

Moisturize as often as you feel your body skin requires it; at least several times a week is recommended. Use body moisturizing lotion after every bath or shower on drier areas of your body, or in winter, when skin tends to be drier. Use the lotion as often and as liberally as you like, except on irritated areas.

A body moisturizing lotion that helps protect your skin from moisture loss is the important third step in your consistent program of total body care.

Your skin needs moisture to function well and look its best, and a body moisturizing lotion helps your skin retain its precious beautifying moisture. Smooth moisturizer over arms, legs, shoulders, torso — everywhere — after your shower or bath for soft, velvety skin.

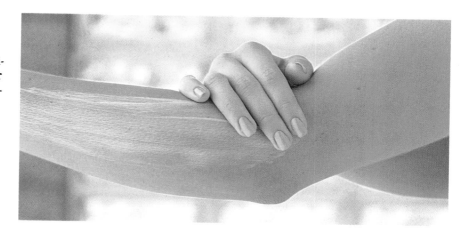

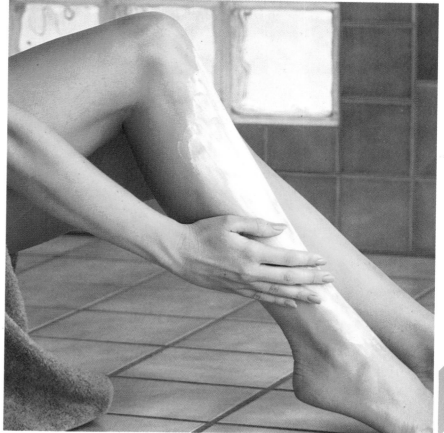

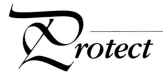

Protect

Heat, cold, environmental dryness, and, in particular, damaging effects of the sun can all contribute to aging skin. To counteract the potential dangers of the environment, you should regularly use a sunscreening lotion with moisturizing agents.

If you engage in active sports or swimming, your sunscreening lotion should be water-resistant and have a sun protection factor (SPF) of at least 10. Whatever your skin type, you need a sunscreen that helps shield your body from the sun's harmful ultraviolet rays and slows down premature aging caused by overexposure. This protective lotion should leave no greasy after-feel.

How and When to Protect Use your sunscreening lotion whenever you are going to be out in the sun. Apply it evenly to clean skin on all uncovered areas of your body. Sunscreen is most effective when you apply it seven to fifteen minutes before going outdoors. Reapply after swimming or strenuous exercise, or if you perspire heavily. Sunscreening lotion may be applied over body moisturizing lotion.

Slow tanning will still occur through a sunscreen. Your body sunscreening lotion functions to help protect your skin from harmful ultraviolet radiation. Even with a sunscreen, however, it's best not to "bake" in the sun for long periods of time, especially between the hours of 10 A.M. and 2 P.M. (11 A.M. to 3 P.M. daylight saving time) when the sun's rays are strongest.

Protecting your skin is the fourth essential step in your all-over, total body skin care. Remember: damage from sun exposure is permanent and irreversible, so it is essential that you include this step in your body skin-care routine.

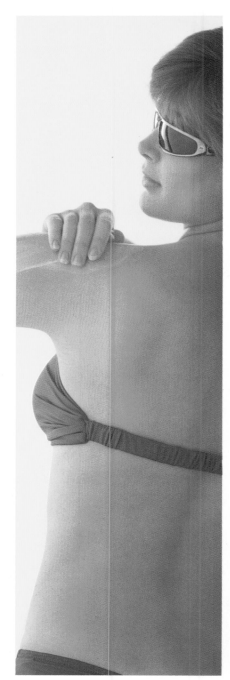

Protecting your skin from the sun's damaging rays is the fourth step in your body-care routine. Smooth **sunscreen** over uncovered skin when you're outdoors, for a softer, younger-looking body.

$\mathscr{Y}$ear-Round Sun Protection

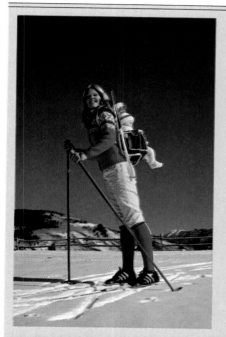

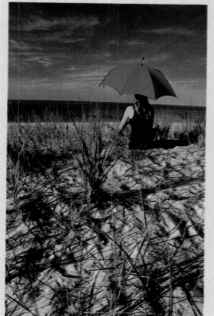

Because your skin is exposed to ultraviolet radiation from the sun whenever you are outdoors, a body sunscreening lotion is important throughout the year, not just on summer days at the beach.

The more distant *winter* sun can be misleading. It's especially important to protect all exposed body skin whenever there is snow — while skiing, ice skating, sledding, or walking, particularly in the mountains where high altitudes intensify the effects of ultraviolet radiation. Snow reflects up to 85 percent of the sun's rays, making the dangers of sun damage even greater in snow conditions than at the beach. In winter, urban areas are also potentially dangerous, as many glass- or mirror-covered buildings reflect sunlight. Use a sunscreening lotion whenever you plan to be outdoors for long periods of time, even in the absence of bright sunshine. Your skin will be exposed to damaging ultraviolet radiation even if the sun isn't shining.

Autumn is a season we are often outdoors, but because the air seems cool, we may not notice prolonged exposure to sunlight. Remember: damaging ultraviolet rays don't feel warm. Use a sunscreening lotion on all exposed body skin whenever you plan to be outside in the fall.

Protection is most critical during the *summer* because the sun is strongest and outdoor activities most popular. Use sunscreening lotion whenever you will be outside: playing sports such as tennis or golf; attending social events such as picnics or barbecues; even gardening or walking to work. If you perspire heavily, reapply your sunscreen often. Even when the sky is hazy, ultraviolet radiation is still strong, increasing the danger of overexposure because you may not be aware of the intensity of the sun's rays. Those who live in high altitudes should take even greater precaution. At the beach, use sunscreening lotion on hazy or sunny days. Sand reflects as much as 17 percent of the sun's rays and intensifies exposure.

Skin damage from sun exposure can occur in the *spring* when the air is still apt to be cool and you do not feel heat rays right away. Protect all exposed body skin with your body sunscreening lotion whenever you plan to be outdoors.

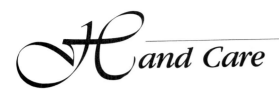and Care

Beautiful hands result from proper, ongoing care. They reflect your commitment to grooming, an unmistakable sign that you pay attention to the details of your appearance. The first step in nail care is correcting minor flaws. Here are some solutions:

Nails that chip, break, peel, or split can be mended with a variety of products available for home use. Nail hardeners, which can be used as a base or top coat, help harden and protect weak, soft nails. However, these must be used with great caution because of their strong chemicals. Discontinue use if you suspect an allergic reaction. Nail wrapping strengthens nails and extends the life of nail polish. Both nail hardeners and nail wrapping give long nails extra protection. To prevent nails from *tearing at the sides,* file only the nail edge to round off the tips.

Ridges can be treated with a special ridge-filling product and a nail-smoothing board. These items even out the ridges as the nail grows out and help prepare the nail surface for polish. (Prominent or new ridges can be symptomatic of an underlying medical problem; consult a doctor.) *White spots,* air spaces in the nail or tiny bruises under the surface, also grow out with the nail. To hide white spots, coat them with opaque nail enamel.

Ragged, uneven cuticles can be prevented by making cuticle care part of your nightly routine. Massage in cuticle conditioner to guard against cracking and drying. Soak your nails weekly in warm, sudsy water, then follow with cuticle conditioner. Next, push back cuticles gently with the rounded end of a manicure stick. Don't trim your cuticles with nail scissors or cuticle nippers; recent evidence indicates that trimming destroys the protective function of the cuticle and can lead to inflammation and infections in the nail bed.

Nail stains can be removed by buffing, which also increases blood circulation. A base coat applied prior to polish helps prevent the enamel color from staining the nail.

You can prevent polish from *bubbling* if you apply it carefully. Make sure your nails are clean, dry, and free of oil, and allow each coat of polish to dry thoroughly. Brush on polish away from direct heat or air-conditioning vents. If polish gets too thick, thin it with a nail enamel thinner. Finally, give freshly polished nails a chance to dry completely. If you don't have time to let them dry naturally, be sure to use a liquid or aerosol drying product.

Tips for Pretty Hands

To protect hands in cold, dry weather, use a rich hand cream with added sunscreen, and always wear gloves outdoors. Carry a purse-sized container of lotion with you and moisturize your hands several times a day.

Since hot water, household cleansing products, and detergents can be extremely drying, wear rubber gloves when you do housework, especially washing dishes. (Keep a pair by the sink to remind you.) For extra moisturization, apply hand cream before putting on gloves.

Heavy work — such as gardening or outdoor chores — calls for heavy gloves to protect skin and nails. Also, if you play golf or racquet sports, try to prevent calluses by wearing the special gloves designed for these purposes.

Always carry an emery board in your purse in case a nail breaks or tears. Rough edges look unsightly and can catch on your clothing.

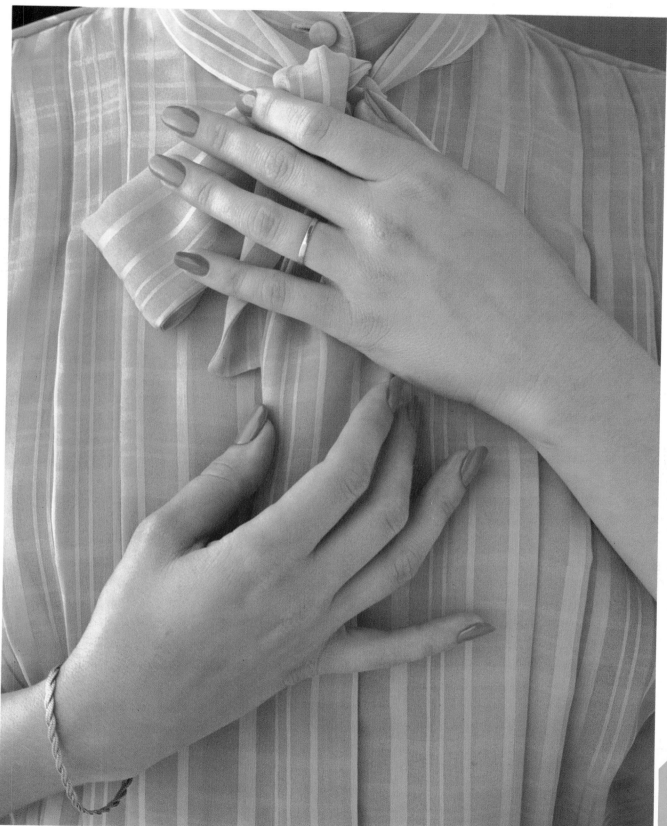

$\mathcal{H}$and Care

Everything you need to take care of your hands is, so to speak, right at your fingertips. Your lifestyle and personal preference affect the length you keep your nails and the shade of polish you choose. However, once you achieve the look you want, maintenance takes just a small amount of time each week. Here's how to give yourself a manicure.

Manicure Tools
Nail polish remover and cotton balls
Emery board
Shallow bowl for soaking your fingertips
Cleansing gel
Clean, soft hand towel
Manicure stick
Cuticle conditioner
Ridge filler and nail buffer (optional)
Base coat, nail polish, top coat
Hand cream

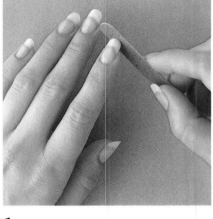

1 Remove old polish with nail polish remover and cotton balls, then file and shape your nails. Use a file instead of nail scissors because cutting can weaken your nails. With an emery board, file your nails in one direction, toward the center. Don't saw the emery board back and forth across the edges of your nails, as this can roughen the surface.

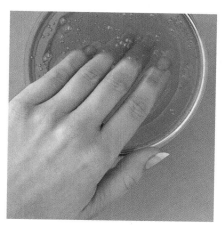

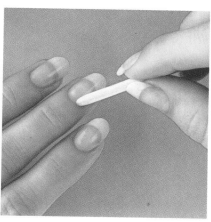

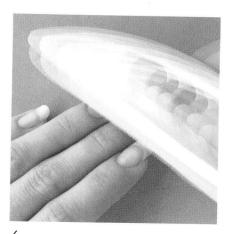

2 Put warm water and cleansing gel into a shallow bowl and soak your fingers for about a minute. As you dry your hands, gently loosen any dirt with a manicure stick.

3 Apply cuticle conditioner along your cuticles. Push back cuticles gently with the blunt, rounded end of a manicure stick. (These sticks are ideal for cuticles and under nails because they are made of soft wood that won't tear or damage the fragile cuticle and under-nail skin.)

4 Depending on your needs, apply ridge filler and/or buff your nails. Always buff nails at an angle in one direction. If you wish to apply polish, remove all traces of cuticle conditioner by patting nails dry with a towel. Nails should be free of oil before you apply polish. Brush on a base coat and allow it to dry. Then apply nail enamel with three quick strokes from the base to the tip — one down the middle of the nail and one on each side. Apply two or three times, allowing each coat to dry between applications. Finish with a top coat; for extra protection, brush it under the tips of your nails. Again, allow it to dry. (You may want to use a special nail-drying product at this time.) To keep hands feeling soft and smooth, rub in hand cream. For extra protection, choose one with added sunscreen.

_F_oot Care

You may not think of including your feet in your regular beauty routine. After all, they're not as visible as the rest of your body. But proper foot care offers many benefits: it completes your head-to-toe beauty look and enhances the appearance of your feet in bare, strappy sandals. It also helps guard against minor foot problems that can leave feet sore or unsightly. Perhaps most important of all, well-cared-for feet make you feel good.

To keep your feet in peak condition, buff and moisturize them regularly. This is especially useful on heels and soles, where calluses are likely to develop. For feet that look and feel sensational, give yourself a pedicure — once a month in cool weather and once every two weeks in warm weather.

Pedicure Tools

Nail polish remover and cotton balls
Toenail clipper
Emery board
Large basin or bowl
Cleansing gel
Pumice stone
Soft nailbrush
Clean, soft towel
Moisturizer
Cuticle conditioner
Manicure stick
Tissue or foam rubber separators
Base coat, nail polish, top coat

Remove old polish with nail polish remover and cotton balls. Trim your toenails with a toenail clipper; refer to the box at left for the proper procedure. Then use an emery board to smooth rough edges and corners.

Put warm water and cleansing gel in a large basin and soak your feet for ten minutes. Use a pumice stone dipped in the water to soften rough skin and calluses. (Regular use of buffing cream in the bath or shower also helps smooth and soften feet.)

With a soft nailbrush dipped in the water, scrub your toenails lightly to loosen dirt and buff your nails. Towel your feet dry.

Apply cuticle conditioner along your cuticles. Push them back gently with the rounded end of a manicure stick. Clean under nails with the pointed end.

If you wish to apply nail polish, separate your toes with tissue or a foam-rubber separator. Begin with a base coat, then follow with two or three coats of polish. (A manicure stick is handy for cleaning smears of polish on the skin around your nails.) Be sure to allow ample drying time between applications. Apply the top coat and allow your nails to dry completely before removing the separators.

Finish by massaging in moisturizer. Begin with your toes, then spread moisturizer over your feet, on your legs, and down again. Rub it well into the soles of your feet.

_T_rimming Toenails

Using a nail clipper, cut each toenail _straight across,_ following the shape of your toe. Toenails should be even with — never longer than — the ends of your toes. But don't cut them too short because the tender flesh under your nails is not meant to be exposed.

Smooth jagged edges with the dark, coarse side of an emery board. Then use the light, fine side to finish smoothing your cut nail edges. Be sure to move the emery board in one direction, toward the center.

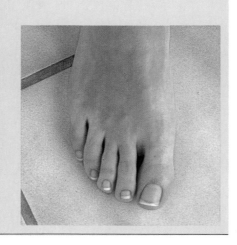

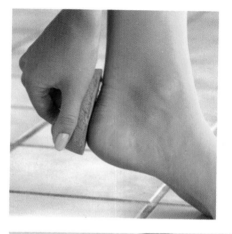

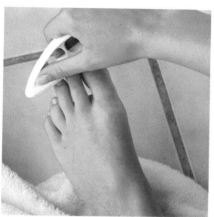

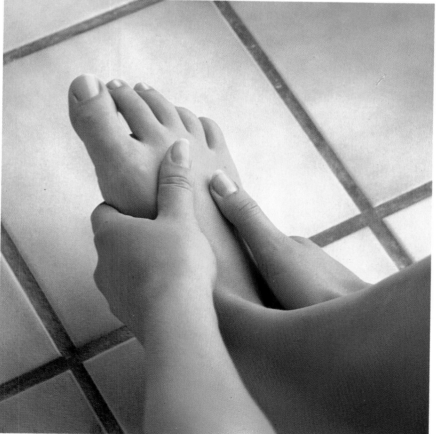

Buy shoes carefully. Check the length and width, and be sure shoes fit well at the heel. Toes should have room to move freely, and uppers should not cause friction when you walk. To get the most accurate fit, shop for shoes at the end of the day when your feet are most swollen. Finally, avoid buying shoes that need "breaking in" — you'll most likely have problems with them later on.

Vary heel heights regularly to help tone calf muscles while soothing heels and soles.

Elevate your feet for a few minutes each day to improve circulation.

Refresh tired feet with a lightly scented talc.

Avoid walking barefoot on hard surfaces; it hardens skin and promotes calluses. However, walking barefoot on sand can be beneficial — sand acts as a natural pumice for your feet.

Body Care

197

*H*air Removal

Hair grows all over the body in varying amounts, distribution, and texture. Your quota of body hair is principally a factor of heredity, but excess growth may in some cases be related to hormonal imbalance or medication. If, as an adult, you notice sudden body hair growth in any area, it's best to consult a physician regarding the cause. Many women are concerned about unwanted hair growth on their legs, under their arms, and on other parts of their bodies. The methods for removing this hair range from professional treatments for permanent removal to home treatments that take it off temporarily or make it less noticeable. Hair removal should be a part of your personal grooming routine; how you accomplish it depends on the area of the body you are dealing with and on your individual needs and preferences.

Electrolysis can be a safe and effective method of permanently removing hair from the body. This technique destroys the hair root through an electric current. A very fine wire needle is inserted into the opening of the hair follicle, and an electric current is transmitted down the needle to destroy the root. Each hair then falls out or is removed with tweezers. Since each hair is individually treated, it takes a long time to remove a lot of hair by this process. Electrolysis may also be costly and uncomfortable, so you should consider it only for removing hair in small areas — your upper lip or chin, between your breasts, or surrounding your navel. Because of possible scarring (if excess current is used) and infection (if equipment is not sterile), it is extremely important to choose a competent professional electrologist. Ask your dermatologist for a recommendation.

Tweezing is a semipermanent method of hair removal. It removes the hair by pulling out the root, and it takes a long time for the hair to grow back. Because it is slightly uncomfortable and tedious, tweezing is not recommended for large areas of body hair, but it may be suitable for stray hairs between your breasts or near your navel, as well as for minor facial hair problems. (Never tweeze hair from a mole or mark on your skin — consult a dermatologist.)

Depilatories — over-the-counter chemical compounds — dissolve or loosen surface hair. You apply a depilatory to your skin, leaving it on for a specified amount of time. When you wipe off the cream, the hair should come off with it. But chemicals strong

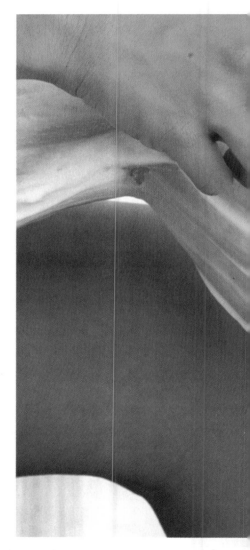

Hair growth on legs and underarms comes off easily with the whisk of a razor when you use body cleansing gel to soften your skin and reduce surface friction. Shaving is one of several grooming options for removing unwanted hair.

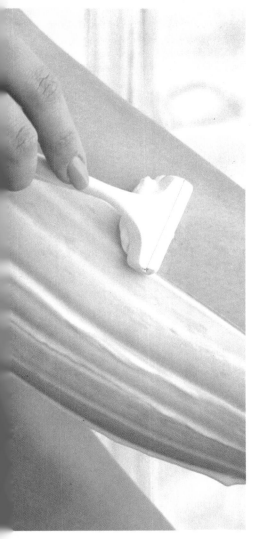

enough to break down the composition of body hair may also irritate your skin. Before you use a home depilatory product, test it on a small, less sensitive area of your body — the tougher skin on your arms or legs. Milder depilatories, specially formulated for hair on the facial skin, are best for this sensitive area. Regrowth after use of a depilatory may take from two to three weeks, although some hairs grow in faster than others.

Waxing is another technique for hair removal that lasts about two to three weeks; it may be less irritating to your skin than chemical depilatories. Warm wax is spread on the area from which hair is to be removed, allowed to dry, then pulled off in hard strips to which the hair adheres. Waxing is suitable for many areas of the body, including the face, and is especially effective for arm, leg, and even underarm hair.

Shaving is the least permanent method of hair removal, since hair may reappear within twenty-four hours. But shaving is an extremely effective and easy method for temporarily removing hair from your lower legs and underarms. A foaming, moisturizing product like body cleansing gel helps a razor glide easily over your skin to remove hair in the bath or shower and helps prevent the dryness that often accompanies shaving. Use of body moisturizing lotion on your lower legs after shaving also helps keep them silky smooth and well conditioned. Your upper thighs and bikini line may not respond well to shaving; regrowth may cause irritation and ingrown hairs.

Bleaching with creams or lotions lightens the color of body hair by chemically lifting the pigment so that the paler color of the hair blends with the skin and is less noticeable. Since bleaching alters the structure of the hair by penetrating the cuticle and tends to make hair coarser, it is best used on only the finest, sparsest growth; also, patch tests are recommended on areas where the product is to be applied to determine whether it will cause irritation. Hair on your arms, legs, and, if needed, bikini line may be bleached effectively. Regrowth of darker roots generally occurs within a week.

Body Care

Pregnancy and You

Hormonal changes that accompany pregnancy affect the way your skin looks and feels, not only on your face but elsewhere on your body. Your skin may become oilier; frequent cleansing with a mild cleansing gel helps. Skin that becomes dry during pregnancy may look and feel less dehydrated through frequent use of body moisture lotion after a bath or shower. Exposure to the sun may cause irregular spotting of body skin during pregnancy, so it is especially important to protect your skin with a sunscreening lotion whenever you are going to be outdoors.

Cholestasis of pregnancy is an itchy condition that results when an increased hormonal level affects the liver. Changes in circulation during pregnancy may cause fine-lined, weblike veins to show through the surface of the skin on your arms, hands, neck, upper chest, or face. These tend to disappear shortly after delivery.

Your body skin may also be affected by physical changes that occur during pregnancy. Because enlargement of the uterus puts pressure on the large blood vessels in the pelvis, veins in the legs sometimes become dilated, and the extremities swell. In some cases, varicose veins develop and persist after pregnancy. To prevent this condition, it is usually recommended that pregnant women keep their legs elevated as much as possible. (If you develop varicose veins, cosmetic surgical treatments are available to remove them.)

Stretch marks are possibly the most prevalent and bothersome of all body skin conditions related to pregnancy. The American Academy of Dermatology estimates that as many as 90 percent of all women develop these marks, which are caused by the pulling and separating of collagen and elastin tissues below the skin's surface, usually on the thighs, buttocks, breasts, and abdomen. Topical creams or oils cannot prevent or help these marks, since the problem originates in the lower layer of the skin. Certain measures may help avoid the development of stretch marks, however; a pregnancy panty girdle helps provide support for the tissues of the abdomen and buttocks, for example, and mild exercises can increase muscle tone in the affected areas. If you develop stretch marks despite your precautions, you may be able to conceal them with body makeup.

Throughout your pregnancy, your personal physician is your best source for all related information. He or she can offer all the advice

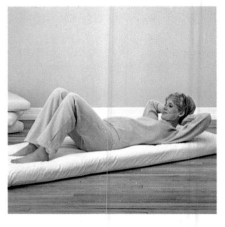

Your pregnancy is a beautiful time in your life — especially when you maximize all the beautifying health benefits of good body care. Now more than ever you'll want to do everything you can for your overall health.

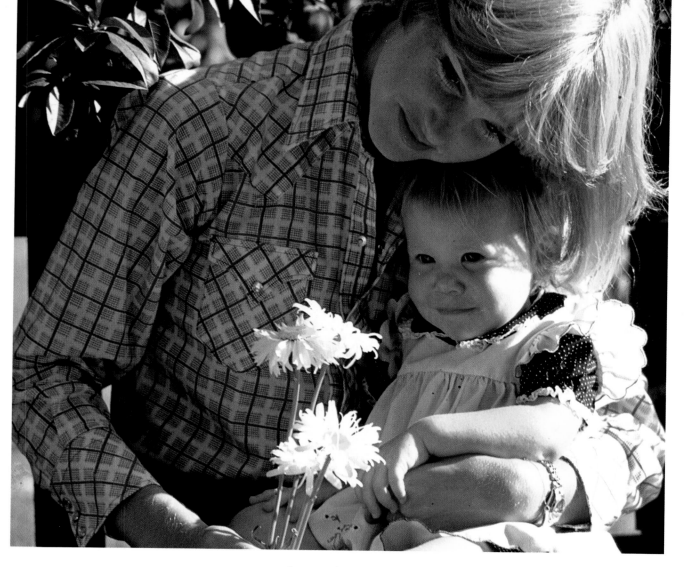

you need regarding your skin's condition, the amount of exercise you need, and the best diet for you. Although an active pregnancy is now considered healthy for many women, it may not be suitable for you individually. Consult your doctor before you begin any type of exercise program or regular sports activity while you're pregnant.

In many cases, pregnancy enhances a woman's beauty, giving her an all-over glow that is characteristic of this very special time in her life. It can be an excellent time to make the most of the way you look and feel, a prime opportunity to take care of yourself and be your healthy best.

Exercise and You

An essential part of total beauty is an overall feeling of well-being — the ability to relax, set priorities, and manage any setbacks. You want to balance the many aspects of your life, to fulfill your responsibilities yet still have time to devote to yourself. Most important, you need to make a commitment to feeling good — physically and psychologically. Specifically, this means developing positive, healthy habits: getting enough sleep, exercising regularly, eating properly. It also means setting goals that are challenging yet realistic.

Exercise There are so many reasons to keep your body in top condition. The most obvious is you'll look sensational. Most likely you'll also feel more energized, be more alert, raise your self-confidence, and be able to handle stress more effectively. And as an extra bonus, you may help reduce your susceptibility to certain diseases. Quite simply, exercise is one activity that guarantees you a return on your investment.

There's an exercise to suit just about every interest, lifestyle, and skill level. Naturally, you'll want to choose something you enjoy, whether it's jogging, swimming, ballet, aerobic dancing, or any of countless other activities. The key is to focus on what you can do, not on what you can't.

Start at a comfortable level and build up gradually; never overdo exercise at the beginning. Keep in mind, however, that for any exercise program to be effective, you must stick with it — vigorously and consistently. When you begin to see results, you'll be encouraged to progress even further.

In addition, you want to make a conscious effort to build movement into your day-to-day activities. Climb stairs. Walk to work, or from the train station or bus stop. Ride your bike to do errands. Bend and stretch when you do everyday household chores. (Be sure to bend your knees when lifting heavy objects to avoid straining your back.) Whenever possible, be a participant rather than a spectator. Once you begin, you'll be amazed at all the opportunities to add exercise to your schedule.

As you set up your individual program, try to combine a number of different exercises and activities. This will work the greatest number of muscle groups and, at the same time, give your routine variety. Aim to include at least twenty minutes of vigorous, sustained

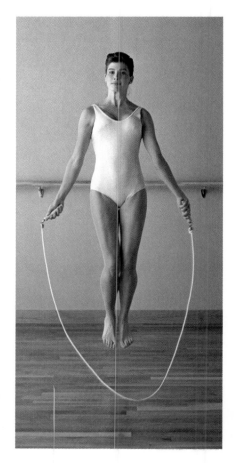

Exercise keeps you trim, fit, and toned — and it makes you feel wonderfully alive. Jumping rope is an excellent aerobic activity that increases circulation and oxygen exchange. This form of exercise can improve your overall strength and stamina and help tone your muscles.

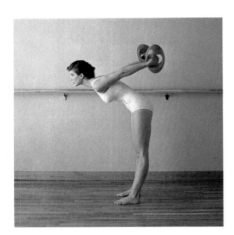

aerobic exercise (activities that increase your oxygen intake and heart rate) at least three times a week: among the possibilities are aerobic dance class, jogging, bicycling, swimming, jumping rope, and cross-country skiing.

To supplement your aerobic workout, you can add sports, spot exercises, and overall stretching to your routine. You'll help firm and tone as you increase your flexibility and coordination. In addition, you might consider joining a health club in your area. Many offer excellent programs for all-around fitness along with such extras as whirlpools, saunas, racquetball and tennis courts, exercise classes, and child-care facilities. No matter what, always check with your doctor before beginning any kind of exercise program.

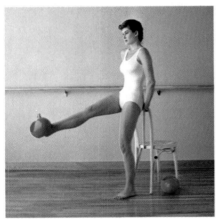

A fit, firm body is worth working for. Weight lifting tones and firms your muscles and improves your coordination and motor skills. Stretching is a mild form of exercise that tones and extends your muscles, strengthens your spine, and increases your flexibility. It can help relieve tension and is excellent for warming up before aerobic exercise or sports.

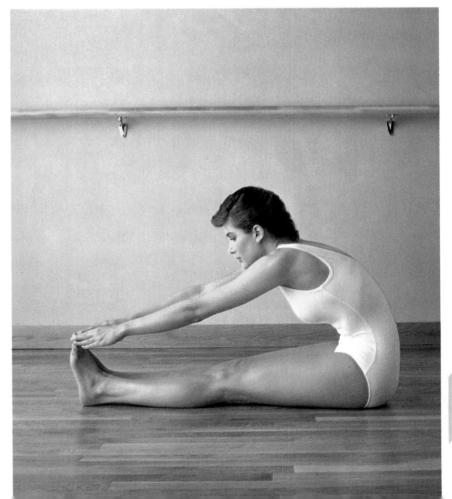

Body Care

Sleep, Relaxation, and You

Sleep You spend about one-third of your life sleeping — so naturally you want to make those hours count. A good night's sleep offers a number of beauty benefits: it can help you feel more alert and alive, it can increase your energy level, and it can make it seem as though you're able to fit more into your day.

How much sleep do you need? Six to eight hours is considered the norm for healthy adults, although your individual needs may vary. And along with the quantity, the quality of your sleep is important. Choose a mattress that gives you the support you need (many experts recommend a mattress that's on the firm side, although you may want to check with your doctor). To elevate the neck properly, one pillow is generally suggested.

Another key consideration is the climate you sleep in. Personal comfort is the first guideline, although some sleep studies indicate the best temperature for sleep is between 64 and 68 degrees Fahrenheit. Avoid rooms that are too dry; mucous membranes can dry out and make breathing more difficult. If dryness is a problem, a humidifier may help, especially in winter.

You'll sleep better, too, if you avoid heavy eating and exercise before bed. Other relaxers include light reading, yoga, and progressive relaxation. And don't overlook the importance of your surroundings. Make your bedroom a comfortable, enjoyable place to be. The best environment for sleep is a room that reflects your personal and very special needs and tastes.

Relaxation No matter how much you fit into your daily schedule, it's essential to work in time for relaxation. Setting aside a few minutes to break from your routine can increase productivity and lift the spirits; it can also help you manage stress.

There is, however, no one relaxation technique that will work for everyone. Some women, for example, may find a leisurely bath, a long walk, or a brisk jog relaxing; others may get the desired results with yoga, meditation, massage, or progressive relaxation. The key is to experiment with different methods — to discover what will refresh *your* mind and relieve *your* tension. Once you find the right activity — or combination of activities — you'll discover the positive effects relaxation can have on your life.

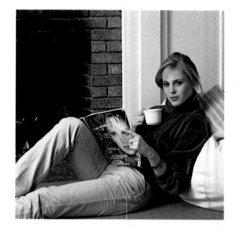

It's important for everyone to take time to preserve interests that are special and provide time alone.

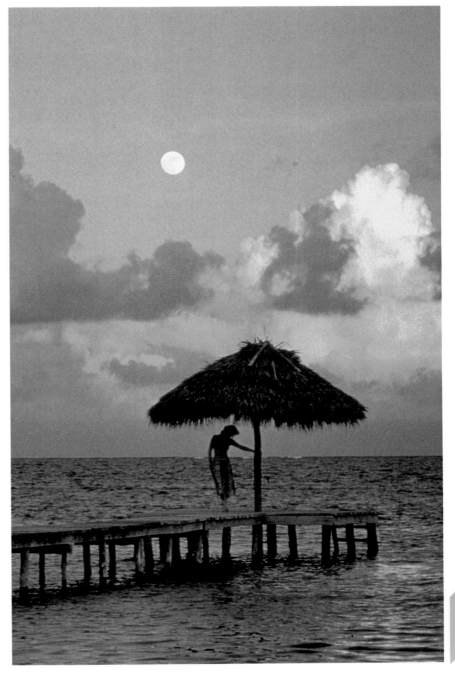

Whether it's an hour's walk on the beach, a hike in the woods, or some pensive time alone in a favorite spot, it's good to get outdoors on a regular basis.

Bathing for Beauty

Taking time to luxuriate in a soothing scented bath is one of the nicest things you can do for yourself. It relaxes your muscles after a vigorous physical workout. It calms your mind after a busy day of responsibilities. And it soaks away tensions to help you sleep better at night or make the transition between a high-pressured day and an elegant evening out. Set an evening aside at least twice a month for a complete beauty bath. Here are some tips for making it a totally luxurious and beautifying treatment.

Begin by setting a relaxing mood for yourself: play your favorite soft music; turn the lights low and light a pretty candle in the bathroom. Have a glass of iced mineral water or club soda handy to sip as you bathe.

Turn on the bathtub faucet and test the water; it should not be steaming hot — which can dry your skin and drain your energy — but warm enough to soothe your body. If you like a scented bath, pour your favorite rich cream bath into the running stream of water. Dry body skin doesn't hold fragrance as long as oily skin, so using a cream bath in your favorite fragrance is a great way to begin layering your scent. For beautiful, foaming bubbles with the merest hint of scent, pour your body cleansing gel under the water tap as it fills the tub.

Before you get into your beauty bath, cleanse your face, following the procedure recommended for your skin type. It's important to remove all soils

and makeup so your skin can benefit from the rising water vapors.

Slip into your bath and remain immersed for at least ten minutes. Relax completely or read a book or favorite magazine as you allow the bathwater and cream bath or cleansing gel to gently clean and soften your body skin.

This is an excellent time to attend to a few beauty tasks: buff elbows and knees thoroughly, applying your buffing cream to areas of rough or hard skin. You might also use a pumice stone on the calluses of your feet and/or shave your legs and underarms, using your cleansing gel to work up a rich lather that makes the razor glide easily over your skin.

A beauty bath is an ideal time to use your facial mask while your skin is clean and your pores are somewhat open from your warm bath. Apply the mask and lie back on an inflatable tub pillow for about ten minutes. (If you're going out afterward, a cool, damp facecloth or damp cotton balls on your eyes refresh and brighten them.) Set a timer for ten minutes so you can relax completely without worrying about how long your mask has been on.

Don't rush your beauty bath — allow at least half an hour to treat yourself to its pleasures and beauty benefits. When you are done, take a quick shower to rinse off your body: if you are planning to go to bed, take a soothing warm shower; if you're going out for the evening, turn the water from warm to cool for an invigorating rinse.

Dry yourself with a clean, fluffy towel. While your skin is still damp, apply moisturizing lotion over your entire body, using a bit extra on dry spots like knees, elbows, and shins. Next, powder yourself all over with talc or dusting powder in your favorite fragrance. If your body moisturizing lotion has just a hint of fragrance, it will not interfere with the powder's fragrance, and the moisturizing lotion helps powder or talc adhere more evenly to your body. Apply powder especially to those areas that tend to perspire most.

Whether you're going to bed or out for the evening, apply some cologne or perfume after your beauty bath. Clean, moisturized skin holds scent well. If you're going out for the evening, scent all your pulse points (see pages 214 and 215).

With your body skin clean, moisturized, and smelling fresh, your tight muscles relaxed, and your tensions soothed, you're ready to apply your makeup for an evening out — or to slip into bed for a restful night's sleep.

Your total beauty bath is a special pleasure you should indulge in whenever you like: in the evening, it can be a pre-bed calmer or a luxurious way to start an elegant evening. It can also be a late-afternoon pickup or a great way to start a day; keep the bath water a bit cooler to refresh and invigorate, or follow your bath with a brisk, cool shower.

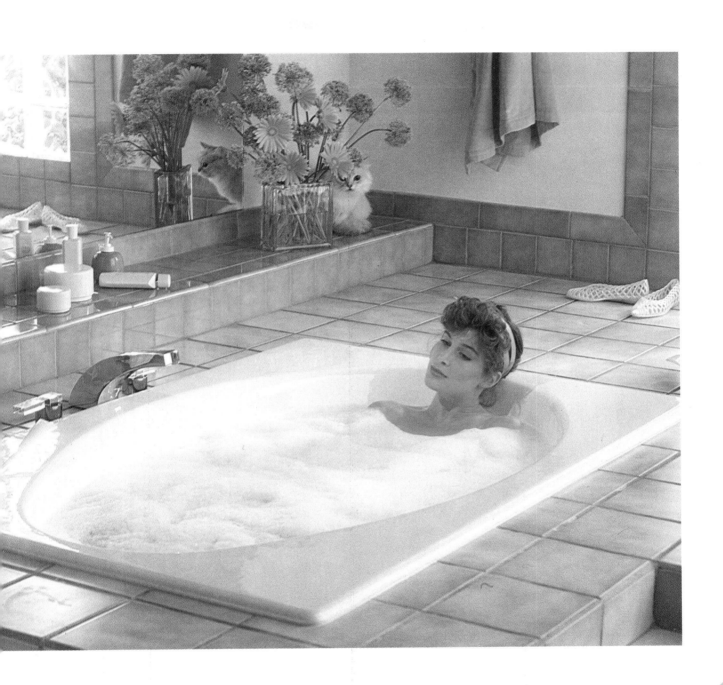

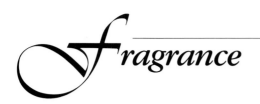

Fragrance

It is estimated that the use of fragrance goes back at least six thousand years. Priests first used perfumes as offerings to the gods; in time, they used them as healing oils. Fragrance later evolved into an element of personal grooming as the nobility of both sexes applied scented oils to increase their attractiveness and allure. But fragrance has never been as popular as it is today.

Formulas for fragrances have been developed over the ages, from simple perfumed oils, to oils blended with alcohol, to today's complex scents. Think of the vast array of aromatic materials that go into a single fragrance: fresh flowers that create soft floral notes; bright citrus scents derived from lemon, orange, and lime; tree moss used to create sensuous mossy tones; spicy notes derived from blending cinnamon, clove, nutmeg, and pepper; rosemary, sage, and basil, which add fresh herbaceous scents; woodsy aromas from sandalwood, cedar, and rosewood; myrrh and fir, which add heady, incenselike scents; even man-made ingredients that simulate natural aromatics. How are these various aromas combined to create the sophisticated perfumes that women use today?

The creation of fragrance is both art and science. Those who blend fragrances are trained scientists with very special talents. The person who assembles a final formula for fragrance is called a master perfumer, or "nose." He or she is trained to distinguish the various combinations of materials that go into fragrances — a skill that takes years of study. During this time the master perfumer also develops an acute and sophisticated sense of smell.

The creator of a fragrance selects ingredients for a fragrance from over five thousand natural and/or aromatic materials. These materials, which come from all over the world, can be extremely expensive. For example, jasmine, which blooms only at night, must be picked within a few hours of blooming, while the petals are still open. Roses must be gathered at sunrise, when they are still moist with dew; four thousand pounds of rose petals are required to make a single pound of the rose oil that goes into a variety of fragrances. Flowers used for floral fragrances must be picked by hand, and it takes one person an entire eight-hour day to pick about fifty pounds of flowers.

Since the eighteenth century, the town of Grasse, in southern France, has been a primary source of flowers for perfume. The warm climate in this area is ideal for growing and harvesting natural jasmine, rose, tuberose, and other flowers used for floral notes in fragrances. During the nineteenth century, when Paris became the fashion capital of the world, prestigious perfume houses were established, and France became famous for its production of fine fragrances. Since then, other countries, including the United States, have found their own distinctive blends of scents to create unique fragrances. Today, fragrances may be made wherever in the world there are materials to create them.

The creation of a fragrance requires a long and careful process of combining many different materials. A fragrance you respond to in a matter of minutes often has taken years to create.

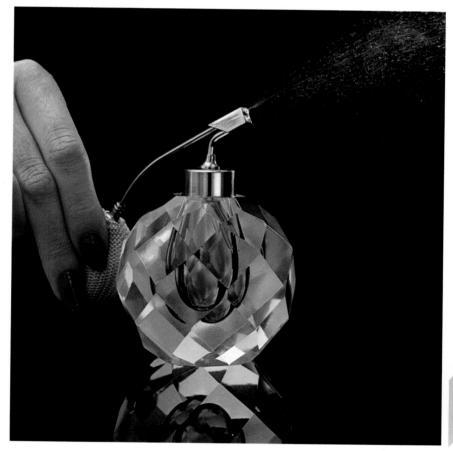

Although fragrance by its nature is ephemeral, it can leave a lasting impression of its wearer. In any single fragrance scores of ingredients combine to create a scent that, when it reacts with your body's chemistry, will become your personal signature.

Taking a Closer Look

Today's woman has an almost infinite variety of moods, personalities, and feelings. And an almost infinite variety of fragrances suits every facet of who you are, how you feel, and how you live.

Fragrances fall into five general categories, according to their composition and aroma. While each type is distinctive and specific, the categories may overlap.

Floral fragrances can be classified as either single floral, fragrances composed mainly of essential oils from one specific flower, or floral bouquets, which blend notes from several different flowers. Within the floral group, some scents are intensely floral, some are notably sweet, and others are very fresh. Both single-floral and floral-bouquet fragrances often express a romantic personality; they're soft and unmistakably feminine.

Greens are fresh outdoor fragrances reminiscent of herbs, leaves, ferns, and freshly cut grass. They are, in fact, composed of many familiar herbs, such as thyme or marjoram, and are usually blended with certain floral oils, such as carnation or lily of the valley. Greens are well suited to active women who spend a great deal of time outdoors; they're naturally fresh and alive.

Aldehydics are exhilarating fragrances that seem to burst with glorious scent. Quite often, they're combined with florals, such as rose or jasmine. Aldehydics — which are classically French — are ideal for the refined, traditional woman; they're distinguished and lend an aura of graciousness.

Orientals are heady, sweet, and exotic fragrances composed of ingredients such as incense, spices, vanilla, and other aromatic substances. They are the strongest and longest lasting of all fragrances. Orientals are for the adventurous and sometimes daring individual; they're bold and warmly mysterious.

Chypres (*SHEE-pruh*) are sophisticated, modern fragrances. Included in this group are combinations and blends of pine, citrus, forest, and mossy notes. Chypres are for the contemporary and fashionable woman; they're rich and always elegant.

Use the five fragrance types as a guide to direct you toward the scents that are most like you, that best suit your personality, moods, and preferences. You may find that more than one fragrance type appeals to you, or that a fragrance type evokes feelings different from those suggested here. This inventory can be a guide to help

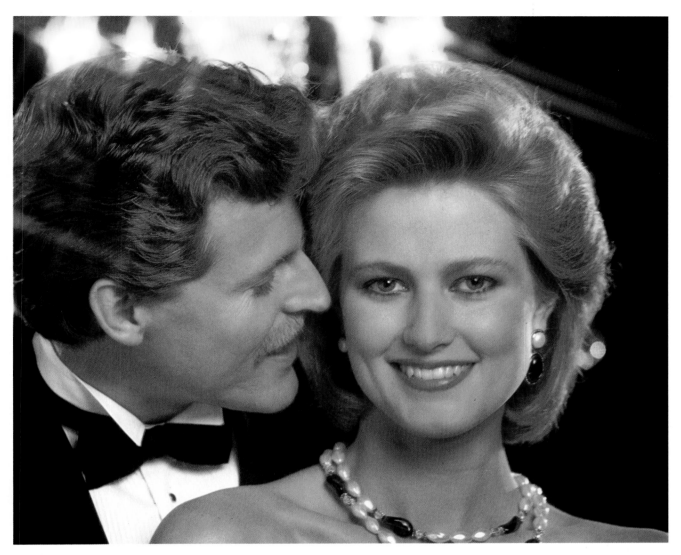

Wonderfully sensuous or whimsically flirtatious, your choices in fragrance create a wardrobe of scent for you to wear — and others to appreciate.

you determine the special combinations of scents that best suit you. Your own preference will be the ultimate determining factor in your choice of fragrance. Also keep in mind that your decision on fragrance can be an emotional one. Certain scents may remind you of a treasured time in your life or a very special place; fragrances have the evocative power to put you in a certain mood or frame of mind.

Because each of us is a composite of many different facets — feminine, exotic, businesslike, playful, maternal, daring — we want to enhance different aspects of our persona at different times in our lives or at different times of day. A wardrobe of fragrances — to suit all the many different women you are, or can be — will enhance all your roles and feelings, and help you make the many transitions in your daily life.

Body Care

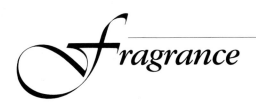
Fragrance

Buying a fragrance is different from buying any other personal item. Purchasing fragrance is an emotional experience, for perfumes can express moods and evoke special feelings and memories. You cannot evaluate fragrances by smelling them in the bottle or admiring their aroma on someone else. You must choose your favorites by trying them on and allowing them to blend with the unique chemistry of your skin oils and moisture.

To test a fragrance, apply a few drops to your inner wrist. Allow them to dry, then pass your wrist back and forth several inches from your nose. The first impression you receive, the most identifiable of the combined scents, is called the *top note*. A fragrance's top note is its brightest — fresh, fervent, and volatile.

Sniff your wrist after ten minutes, holding it close to — but not touching — your nose. As a fragrance begins to blend with your body chemistry, the essence reaches its deepest intensity. The second impression you receive is of the *middle note,* the mellow heart of the fragrance. At this point you can decide whether you like the impression of the fragrance.

You may not notice the lingering *bottom note* of a fragrance until two to three hours after you apply it. Bring your inner wrist up to your nose and inhale deeply. This — the final impression, generally composed of wood, moss, or musk scents — is of the aroma those around you will smell. In some fragrances these three stages may not be noticeable, but in others they will be obvious.

Sample fragrances in midmorning, when your sense of smell is most accurate, and at least several hours after eating, for spicy foods can alter your sense of smell. Since it is difficult to evaluate a great variety of scents at the same time, limit your selection to two possibilities, sampling one fragrance on each wrist.

Your selection of a fragrance should be based on your evaluation of how it suits your personality, your moods, and your preferences. The most important factor in buying fragrance, however, is how well you like the way a particular scent reacts with your unique body chemistry. The same fragrance never smells the same on any two women, so you can choose a fragrance and make it yours. And don't limit yourself to a single selection. Build a wardrobe of fragrances for all the moods and occasions in your life.

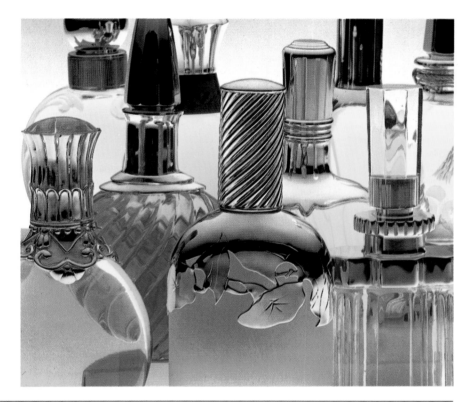

Fragrances not only smell wonderful, they come in elegant, beautiful bottles. Display yours in a convenient location so they're always within reach.

ℳaking Sense of Scents

Once you've chosen your favorites, how much of these fragrances you should wear depends on the kind of impact you want to make, the mood you wish to impart, the ambience of scent you want to surround you. Subtle and fleeting? Direct and dramatic? Mysteriously atmospheric? Your choice may depend on the time of day, your mood of the moment, the occasion, or the people you'll meet.

Fragrance strength may depend on the *type* of scent you select (Oriental scents are the most powerful and longest lasting), but it also depends directly on the form of fragrance you use.

Of all the liquid forms of scent, **perfume** has the highest concentration of fragrance oil in ratio to the alcohol with which it is blended. The most expensive form of fragrance, perfume is the strongest and dressiest, and it lingers longest. A touch of perfume at pulse points will surround you with scent when you want to feel ultrafeminine.

Eau de toilette in the French tradition ranks second in strength, as more alcohol and sometimes water are used to dilute the fragrance oils; with its greater proportion of alcohol, eau de toilette evaporates more quickly over time. You may want to use more of it over your body skin for immediate fragrance impact, but you'll need to reapply eau de toilette throughout the day or evening to keep your scent fresh and strong. Eau de toilette is a versatile form of fragrance that's just right when you want a long-lasting fragrance for an active lifestyle.

Cologne in the French tradition — which has the lowest ratio of fragrance oils to alcohol and water — is the most fleeting liquid form of scent. Cologne may be splashed or sprayed on lavishly, but you'll need to repeat applications often if you want continuous, all-day fragrance. With its minimal lingering power, cologne is appropriate for your moods, occasions, and roles that call for light scents. Just the right touch for your business or daytime image, cologne can be reapplied for extra impact after five.

Scented bath products — soaps, powders, talcs, lotions, and milk baths — provide just a hint of soft fragrance. They are intended for your quietest, most subtle fragrance needs or as basic underlayers for more intense forms of fragrance.

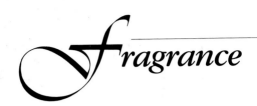

Fragrance

There are as many reasons to wear fragrance as there are ways to wear it. A fresh, lighthearted fragrance can lift your spirits just when they need it. A spray of the right scent can make you feel romantic, feminine, and sensuous. Fragrance can evoke mystery or add drama. It can make you feel luxurious and elegant or winsome and lively. Fragrance creates an impression that becomes part of your total beauty. You can wear one fragrance so only a single scent is clearly identified with you. Or you can experiment with a variety of fragrances to suit your mood or the occasion.

Choose your fragrance with the same careful thought you apply to your wardrobe. Use a fresh, bright, sporty fragrance for days when you're dressed casually, then switch to a dramatically intense scent when you dress up in the evening.

Layer your fragrances to increase their holding power and create different impressions of scent as the day or evening wears on. Start with a rich cream bath fragrance in your bathwater, then puff on matching talc or dusting powder. Spray the same fragrance of cologne under the hair at the back of your neck, on your shoulders, and at your waist. Then dab on matching perfume at pulse points: your inner wrists, behind your ears, behind your knees, at the base of your neck, and inside your elbows. Carry a purse-sized spray cologne or perfume with you for touch-ups during the day or evening.

Use your fragrances creatively. Make a sachet by saturating a cotton ball with your favorite fragrance and place it in a closet or dresser drawer. Fragrance can also be sprayed on dried flower arrangements or in lined dresser drawers to add a whisper of scent to linens. Place empty bottles in lingerie drawers to add a delicate scent to your underclothes.

Fragrance is the ideal way to be good to yourself, to make yourself feel special — and let others know you're special. Wear it to enhance your mood, to express who you are, what you like, how you feel. Make fragrance a part of your personal beauty statement every day — the finishing touch to a perfectly groomed and totally beautiful you.

A drop of fragrance behind your ears, a gentle stroke at the base of your throat, on your wrists, inside your elbows, or behind your knees — your pulse points are where your skin's chemistry combines beautifully with fragrance to surround you with sensual aromas.

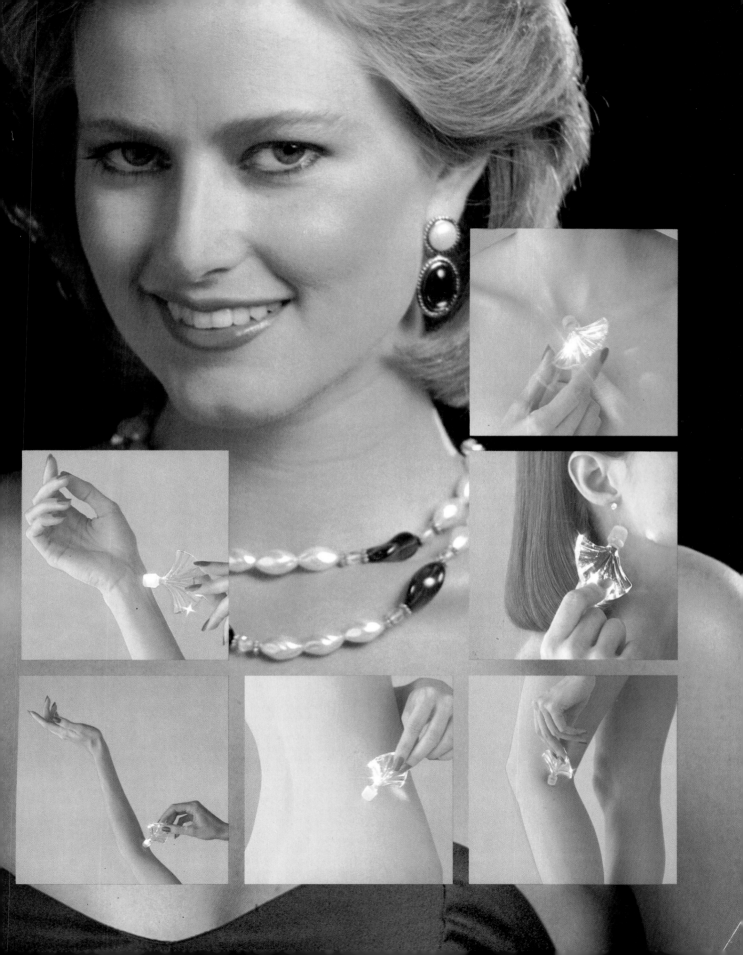

ℱashion Sense

Your wardrobe, like your makeup, says a lot about you. It reflects your tastes, your moods, your way of life, and, of course, your personal style. The way you acquire — and store — your wardrobe is equally revealing. Consider the inside of your closet, for example. How it looks often indicates how well organized you are. There's also your shopping habits. Does the sight of a sale rack excite you, or does it leave you feeling weak in the knees? Do you come home from a shopping spree with just what you needed, too many items, or just a migraine headache?

Choosing a wardrobe that suits your individual style and needs is a skill worth developing. The following pages include information on three important elements: organizing your closet, shopping tips, and how to select clothes that are most flattering to your figure.

When it comes to organizing your closet, the key word is *discipline*. Go through it piece by piece, putting items in the following groups:
• Those to give away. This includes clothes that don't fit, are out of style, or that you haven't worn in the last year (two years maximum!). Remember that the value of clothes you give to a charitable organization is tax-deductible; be sure to get a receipt.
• Those that need dry cleaning, laundering, or altering. Don't keep anything in your closet that isn't in top condition. As a general rule, you shouldn't alter any item you're not sure you're going to keep. Although altering is less expensive than replacing a garment, it can still be costly.
• Those items you wear. Hang similar items together — blouses, dresses, slacks, jackets, skirts, and so on (separate suits and two-piece outfits). Check to see that everything is hung straight; fasten zippers and buttons and, if possible, use wood, plastic, or padded hangers to give garments extra support. Lay sweaters and knits on shelves or in drawers or boxes; hanging can stretch the neckline and shoulders.

It's important to leave ample room between garments in your closet and to avoid hanging one item over another. Clothes that have room to "breathe" last longer, and articles are less likely to wrinkle. If you're short on space, consider these closet extenders:
• A second bar, hung at about waist height. (You may have to adjust your existing bar accordingly.)
• Multiple blouse, skirt, or pants hangers, which can accommodate up to six pieces each.
• Clear plastic storage boxes for sweaters, gloves, scarves, belts, socks, and other unhangables.

Now that you're organized, it's time to look closely at the items in your wardrobe. Chances are you'll find certain gaps, and by adding a specific item you can create a terrific new outfit. You may also discover that your clothes may not suit your current lifestyle. If you've started a new job recently, for example, your wardrobe may require a more professional look. Or perhaps you're short on items for a particular season: you've got dozens of T-shirts but no winter sweaters. Whether you're looking for one special item or a complete wardrobe overhaul, you'll find these shopping tips can help save both time and money:
• Do your homework. Make a list of what you have, as well as things you want to buy. Set up a realistic budget, deciding in advance how much you want to spend on specific pieces. Read the fashion magazines to get general ideas; then study your local newspaper to find out what's available at stores in your area.
• Try different types of stores. Each has its own specialty. Department stores, for example, generally carry wardrobe basics. The selection is large and prices are usually moderate. Department stores also usually offer advantages such as liberal return policies, regular sales, a good range of clothes, and availability of charge accounts, catalogues, and shopper services.

In small boutiques you'll most likely find unique merchandise and personalized service. Shop at these small stores for very new, high-fashion items, but be ready for higher price tags.

At women's specialty stores, there's usually a wider selection of clothing for a variety of needs and occasions. Most specialty shops project a distinct image; you'll feel most comfortable and have the best luck at those where the style matches your own.

Shop at designer discount shops and outlets for low prices, but be prepared for a limited selection, minimal service, and strict return policies. Make sure to check each garment for flaws, and be sure the item fits you well.

• Take advantage of professional advice. A good sales person knows the merchandise and offers assistance, gives you an honest opinion, and never is intimidating or applies high pressure. When you've found a good one, get her card and introduce yourself. Ask for her on future shopping trips and request that she call you when new items arrive, at sale time, or before fashion and trunk shows.

You may also want to shop at stores that offer special fashion consulting or shopper services. You may give the store consultant a budget, and she will put together a mix-and-match wardrobe suited to your individual needs; or the consultant may come to your home and do a wardrobe evaluation, followed by a recommendation of articles to purchase. These

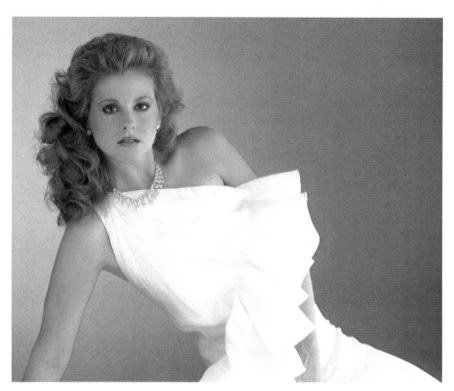

services can be extremely beneficial, but find out in advance whether there's a fee or minimum purchase required.

• Don't limit your shopping. If you're petite, shop the boys' department for designer-label shirts, sweaters, and blazers at much lower prices. Don't automatically pass by the designer section. You may find you prefer one fabulous item in place of several less expensive ones, or you may run across a not-to-be-missed sale item. And even if you can't afford to buy, you can always get ideas of what to look for — especially important if you're an outlet shopper.

• Be a smart shopper. The time you shop makes a difference; stores are usually less crowded early in the week, during the morning hours, and in early evening. For serious shopping, eliminate Saturdays; also, if possible, avoid buying when you need something to wear the same night.

When you shop, it helps to look and feel your best. But be sure to

wear comfortable shoes (carry heels in your bag if you're trying on dressy clothes) and garments that are easy to take on and off. And if you're looking to match up a specific item, take it or a fabric swatch with you.

Before making a purchase, double-check for proper fit; a three-way mirror is best. Also read the care instruction labels; if something needs to be dry cleaned or hand washed, be sure you're willing to spend that time and money. Finally, take a close look at the fabric, lining, seams, zipper, buttons, and so on, especially if the item is on sale.

• Ask yourself questions. Is the color flattering? Does it go with other things in your wardrobe? Does it fit your lifestyle? Can you afford it? Is it a good style for your figure? Be honest. To help you find clothes well suited for you, read over the guidelines on pages 218 to 221.

Fashion Sense

Begin by taking a scrutinizing look at yourself, without any clothes on, in a full-length mirror. Pinpoint the parts of your body you think should be improved. Diet, exercise, and posture can help you correct many, but not all, figure problems. Problems that can't be improved by diet or exercise, however, may be improved with the proper clothes.

In addition to finding what you don't like about your body, acknowledge your strong points. If you have good shoulders, delicate wrists or ankles, a small waist, a well-proportioned bustline, or nicely rounded hips, you can play them up with your clothes. The guidelines that follow will help you select clothing that _enhances_ the beauty of your body.

A _short neck_ appears to look longer when you wear open necklines; a V-neck both slims and elongates your neck — the narrower and deeper the V, the better. Long necklaces, even to your waistline, worn over any style top also help. Always wear the top buttons of shirt collars open, and try jackets with long, slim lapels that button at the waist or hipbone. Long rectangular scarves, knotted or tied at your bustline, can also create an elongated neck look. Also experiment with low-cut and off-the-shoulder styles — worn with long necklaces.

A _long neck_ may give you a graceful, swanlike look, but try wearing higher collars with a ruffle detail or Victorian-style high-buttoned collars. Turtlenecks and bulky cowls are also flattering, as well as shirts buttoned to the top. High, rounded necklines topped with choker-style necklaces or small silk squares knotted at the neck make a long neck look shorter.

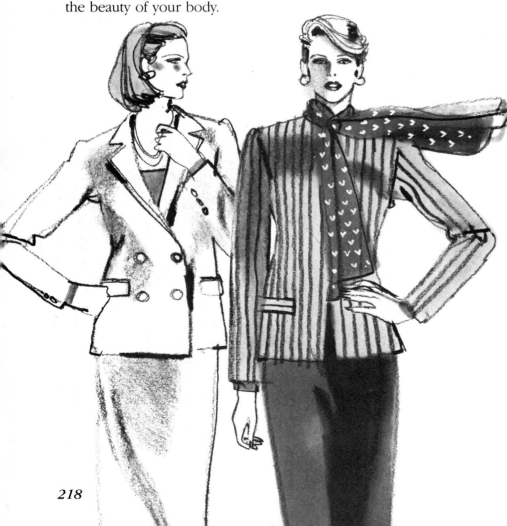

Narrow or sloping shoulders can be made to appear broader and/or squarer by the use of shoulder pads. Boat-neck tops help increase the horizontal line of your shoulders, and nipped-in waists with dark bottoms add width to your upper body. In some cases, blouses with puffy sleeves give volume to your shoulders, and peasant blouses with elasticized necklines — worn so they graze your upper arms — create a more horizontal look for shoulders.

Wide shoulders can be an attractive asset when you square them nicely so your clothing falls well. But you can add roundness by drawing attention inward with neck detail — V-necks, scoopnecks, or soft bows. Sleeveless shifts or tank-top styles only exaggerate wide shoulders, while looser shift sleeves worn to mid-upper-arm length or longer help diminish shoulder size. Avoid styles with shoulder seams; softer looks such as dolman sleeves also add curves. And bright, wide skirts give proportion to the overall look.

A thick waist can be minimized by layering effects. Keep belts narrow (one inch is the best width) but not too skinny, and wear a loose-fitting vest, cardigan, blazer, or jacket with waist-shaping darts over belted separates or dresses. For skirts, choose dirndls or A-lines with wide waistbands. Pants with gathered, slightly pleated waists can shape your hips. Extended shoulders also appear to narrow your waist.

A short waist can be made to look longer by dresses with dropped waistlines that flare somewhat at hipbone level. Also try blouses, shirts, and sweaters worn over skirts or pants, loosely belted with a narrow belt at your hips. When you tuck in shirts, blouse them out at pants or skirt waistline (tuck in tightly, then lift arms overhead) to conceal a short waist. Try straight-line tunic tops too.

A long waist can be improved by high- or wide-waisted skirts and pants and dresses with waistlines slightly above your natural waist. Mid-knee lengths in skirts add length to your legs and shorten your upper body, while longer-length pants create a similar effect. Experiment with wide belts and try leather or fabric sashes tied just above your waist.

Shapeless, skinny, or heavy arms are best concealed in blousy sleeves and bulky, loose-fitting, long-sleeved sweaters for winter and flowing, sheer-fabric blouses for warmer weather. Dark silk or translucent blouses with large, voluminous sleeves that flow over arms are great for dressy occasions, and gauzy peasant blouses or long sleeves rolled to mid-forearm are attractive for casual days.

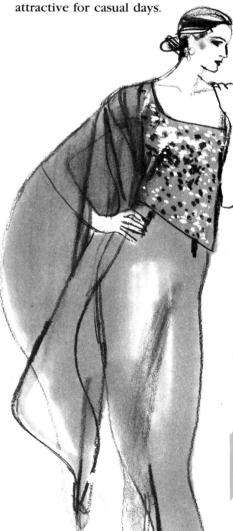

Fashion Sense

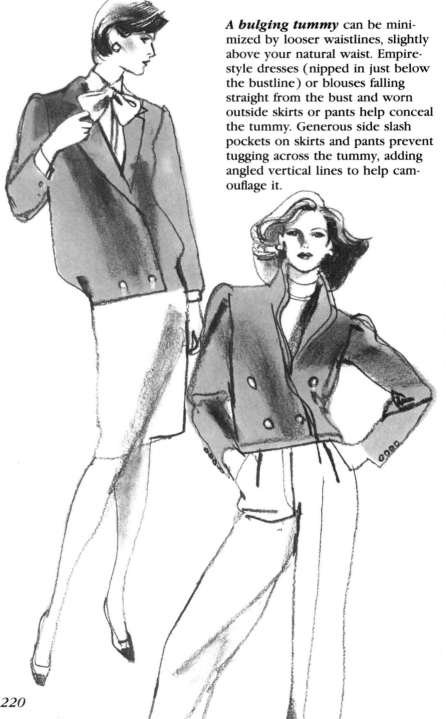

A bulging tummy can be minimized by looser waistlines, slightly above your natural waist. Empire-style dresses (nipped in just below the bustline) or blouses falling straight from the bust and worn outside skirts or pants help conceal the tummy. Generous side slash pockets on skirts and pants prevent tugging across the tummy, adding angled vertical lines to help camouflage it.

Wide hips are best corrected by keeping lines straight and vertical from shoulder to hipbone level; try vests, cardigans, jackets, and blazers that graze your hips. Too much detail at your waist, even if it's small, can widen the look of your hips. Softly gathered, wide, and loose waistbands are best; wear them with narrow, loose belts and full tops loosely tucked in. Straight, shift-style dresses with extended shoulders also help minimize hips.

Straight, narrow hips can acquire curves from clothing with lots of detail at the waist. Pretty, wide belts in contrasting colors or bright metallics that cinch in your waist give extra dimension to thin hips. Gathered and fitted waistlines on shirts and pants add roundness to the hips, as do full, peasant-style skirts with snug waistbands.

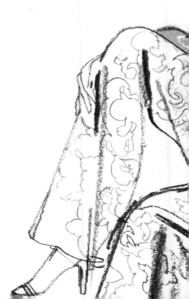

A big bottom is best concealed with full or loosely fitting skirts without accented waistlines. Wear well-cut, tailored pants that are not too tight. Long, straight-cut vests, cardigans, blazers, and jackets cover your derrière loosely to diminish its size. Straight, shift-style dresses with lots of hip room and extended shoulders also help.

A flat bottom can be corrected by belting loose tops over pants or skirts and blousing up the fabric above, and especially below, the waistline. Snug-fitting waistlines with gathers or pleats round out your bottom, as do wide belts that cinch in your waist over bulky and full skirts and pantaloon-style pants.

Tall figures should pay attention to hemlines; depending on proportionate leg length, skirts should reach mid-kneecap to just below the knee — shorter lengths add height to the overall look. Full, soft lines in dresses and separates diminish height, and contrasting colors in separates with accented waistlines also help shorten a taller figure. Wear clothes with horizontal accents such as wide belts and horizontal stripes or patterns and bold prints in small designs that add a busy look, diminishing body length.

A short figure looks best in separates of compatible tones or the same colors, with minimal waist and neck detail; wear shirt collars open and avoid fussy, high necklines. Hemlines should be right at the middle or bottom of the kneecap. Pants should never be shorter than anklebone length. Simple high-heeled pumps with dark or vertically striped stockings, or delicate sandals with skin-tone stockings, add length to legs. Keep clothing lines vertical and elongated, using vertical stripes and patterns; jackets, blazers, cardigans, or vests should be short, hitting at the waist or just below. All accessories — belts, purses, scarves, jewelry — should be proportionately small, not overwhelming. Play up your more delicate figure with small, dainty accents.

An overall large frame looks smaller in darker solids; use bold colors in small accessories like belts or scarves. Keep patterns simple — large geometrics or little, busy designs accentuate larger frames — and avoid extremes in hemlines or pants length. Try to entice the eye inward with decorative belt buckles, detailed lapels on jackets or blazers, and necklaces with pendants worn just below the hollow of the throat. Proper fit at shoulders, waist, and hips is essential.

An overall small frame looks more impressive in bright or light solids worn with neutral, small-sized accessories. Too-short or too-long skirt hemlines should be avoided. Pants should be slightly long, with fitted waists, to add dimension to your figure. Wear horizontals such as boat-neck and off-the-shoulder styles. Clothes should fit perfectly all over and perhaps have slightly extended shoulders. Avoid prints, patterns, and stripes; they tend to overwhelm the smaller frame. Shoes and stockings should be simple, in neutral shades.

$\mathcal{P}$utting It All Together

Jennifer is a homemaker and mother with two small children to care for. Her days are full of responsibilities; they start early and are busy throughout. Jennifer's beauty routine must be streamlined, since she has little time to herself. She wants a fresh and natural, healthy and youthful daytime look. With a tight schedule in which care of her family is the top priority, she likes to save time on beauty care without cutting important corners.

Since her *skin* is oily, Jennifer has to cleanse it in the morning as well as at night. She uses her mask every other day as part of her evening cleansing routine to keep oiliness under control. After her regular cleansing and masking, Jennifer uses a protecting liquid foundation to help reduce shine on her facial skin. She then applies basic daytime *makeup*: translucent face powder in a light peach shade; brown eyebrow pencil to match her coloring; a medium plum eye shadow on her lids with a pale, pearly pink highlighter on the browbone; a brown eyeliner and mascara; and a soft coral lip color. Jennifer's morning skin-care and makeup routine takes a total of fifteen minutes and gives her a fresh, soft look all day — with just a few touch-ups of lip color. For evenings out, Jennifer adds a darker plum eye shadow for contour, applies a contour blusher shade under her daytime blusher, and a brighter coral tone to her lips.

Jennifer wears her *hair* shoulder length because she likes the versatility of wearing it down at night and up and away from her face during the day. Because her hair tends to be oily she washes it every day, conditioning just the ends to prevent tangling. Jennifer's hair is thickly distributed, fine in texture, and very straight — an ideal combination for shoulder-length hair — and she allows it to dry naturally after washing. Before evenings out, Jennifer uses an intensive conditioner on the bottom half of hair shafts to protect them and make them extra shiny. After it dries she puts her hair in electric rollers to add elegant volume with curls.

Jennifer's two calisthenics classes a week help keep her *body* toned, and for fun and relaxation she plays tennis with a friend at least once a week for ninety minutes. Her choice of fragrances suits her romantic personality and is based on floral notes. For daytime she likes to express a joyful mood with green fragrances; for evenings out she likes the elegance of chypres. The basis of Jennifer's

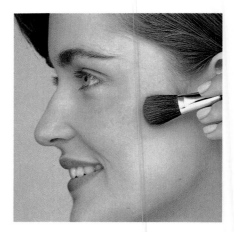

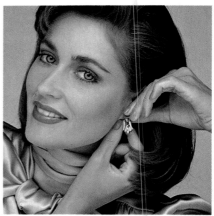

Jennifer's busy schedule demands a beauty routine that's efficient and effective. Her morning regimen takes just fifteen minutes, and she's ready for the day's many activities.

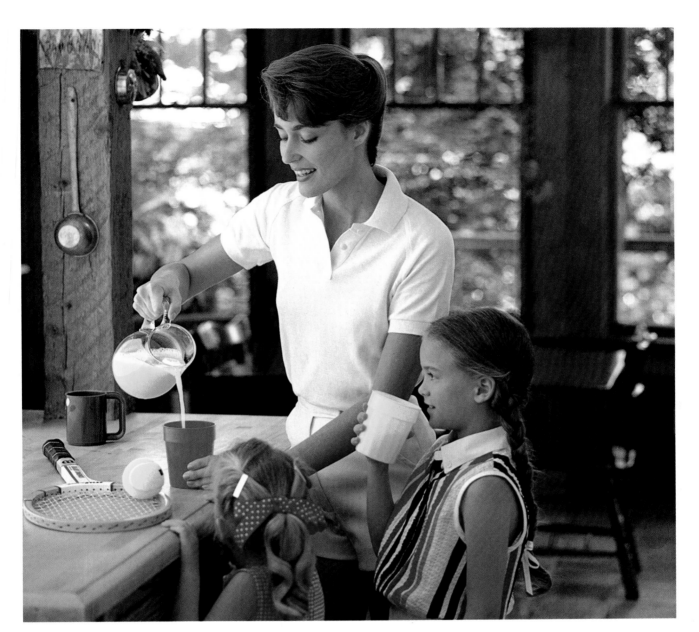

wardrobe is casual daytime wear, with dressier clothes for evening. Turtleneck tops and sweaters help make her neck appear shorter, and skirts with gathered waistlines, hemmed at mid-knee, add desired shape to her bottom while diminishing her height. For evening, Jennifer chooses a romantic style: high-necked, ruffled blouses or dresses and full skirts with a great deal of detail at her waist.

Beauty musts: keeping skin and hair clean to control oiliness; using versatile makeup and hair-styling techniques for quick day-to-evening transitions; protecting her skin with sunscreen when she's out of doors, especially playing tennis; and at least once a week, an evening beauty bath after a hectic day.

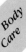

Body Care

223

$\mathcal{P}$utting It All Together

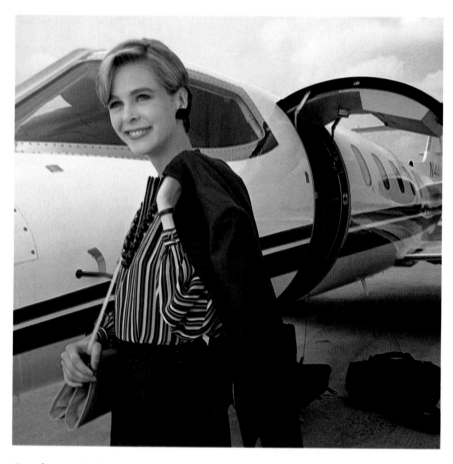

Carol, a career woman on the go, needs a beauty routine that's well organized. To achieve the professional look she needs every day, her morning beauty routine emphasizes glamour makeup.

Carol is a single career woman who travels frequently. She needs time in the morning to put together a sophisticated business look, so she adjusts her beauty routine with trade-offs — a short, simple hairstyle gives Carol more time for makeup, and a superorganized wardrobe helps her make efficient choices when she's in a hurry.

Carol's dry *skin* needs extra protection because she spends so much time in the dehydrating atmosphere of airplanes. She moisturizes daily and always uses sunscreen, knowing she will be outdoors at least part of every day. After applying a creamy, protective foundation, Carol begins her *makeup* routine with translucent face powder and a cream cheek color to accent her cheekbones, then applies a soft berry tone blusher. For sophisticated daytime eyes,

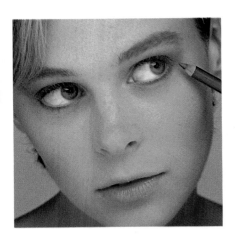

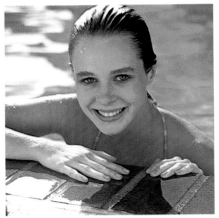

Carol uses the Starlit look from the Glamour Adventure, using deep green and pale brown eye shadow with a teal eye-defining pencil. For lip color, she uses a lip pencil in a red tone, filling in with a bright rose, then adds lots of gloss. For evenings out, she touches up her blusher by using a more intense tone over her daytime shade, and adds a paler green eye color tone to her inner eyelid for Dazzle eyes. She gives her evening lips extra dimension by first lining them, then using a darker rose shade on her top lip and a lighter, brighter tone on her bottom one.

Carol keeps her naturally blond *hair* short in a soft style that flatters her oval face. She brightens the color of her dry hair with professional highlighting, so she needs a regular conditioner every time she washes her hair and an intensive conditioner after every other shampoo. The conditioners help hold moisture and shine in Carol's hair when she styles it with a blow-dryer after washings. She uses decorated combs to pull one side of her hair back for dressy evenings.

Carol takes extra care to apply moisturizer all over her *body* every day. She also finds regular aerobic exercise essential to developing the stamina she needs every day. Jogging thirty minutes at least three times a week is ideal for her lifestyle, since she can do it anywhere, even when she travels. She also swims as often as she can. Carol favors spicy scents that convey her adventurous personality: for daytime she wears the fresh scent of green fragrances; for evening she prefers the mysterious mood created by Oriental fragrance notes. To give needed volume to her upper body and bustline, Carol's daytime business fashion is full-shaped blouses in light, bright colors and slimmer-cut skirts, nipped at the waist. She keeps her skirt lengths at mid-knee and jackets just below her waist to give her legs a more elongated look. For evening Carol finds that puffy sleeves and narrow skirts worn with bright belts and high-heeled sandals add dimension to her bustline and length to her legs.

Beauty musts: moisturizing and protecting her dry skin to keep it fresh and dewy; simple hair styling that allows plenty of time for morning makeup; regular aerobic exercise for added energy; and layering fragrance to make it last.

Body Care

$\mathcal{P}$utting It All Together

Gail is a working mother who runs a consulting business from her home. She works from early morning until midafternoon, when her children come home from grade school. Since her life is varied and busy, with many professional and household responsibilities, Gail schedules different elements of her beauty routine throughout the day.

Gail's **skin** is normal in type and light in tone, so she puts effort into maintaining its condition with regular skin care that emphasizes sunscreen protection. Since Gail's time with her children is often spent outdoors, she uses a sunscreen under her makeup every day. Her **makeup** needs vary from a natural, easy look for home, to the professional polish she needs for business appointments, to a dressier appearance for evenings out. After freshening her skin and protecting it (with sunscreen and foundation) in the morning, Gail uses the Glamour Basics daytime look to start the day. Before business appointments she adds the sophistication of contouring effects with a pink blusher to give more definite angles to her cheeks and reduce their width; Gail blends highlighter into her foundation at the top of her cheekbones, strokes blusher on under the highlighter and a contour blusher under the lighter shade, blending it to her hairline. For a sophisticated daytime eye look, she brings her basic blue lid color down under her eye to the lower lash base and adds a deeper green for contour in the crease, between the blue lid shade and an ivory highlighter on the brow-bone. To make her eyes appear larger, she extends the medium blue lid color slightly beyond the outer corner of her eyes and outlines top and bottom lids with a blue eye-defining pencil. She outlines her lips with a deep-toned lip pencil, filling in with a medium russet lip color, then whisks on a glimmer of gloss.

For her evening look, Gail uses the same basic techniques that work for her business look but brightens the colors; the pink blusher is changed to a more intense berry tone for cheeks, and instead of the blue, green, and ivory eye shadows, she tries a smoky effect with brown, moss green, and almond highlighter. She changes the russet lip color to a deep, bright spice for evenings.

Gail wears her **hair** medium length, allowing her to style it in a way that is most flattering to her square jawline. She sometimes pulls her hair back at her ears with combs, a style ideal for both

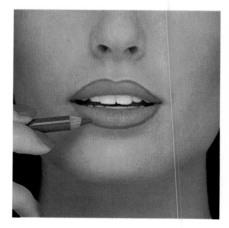

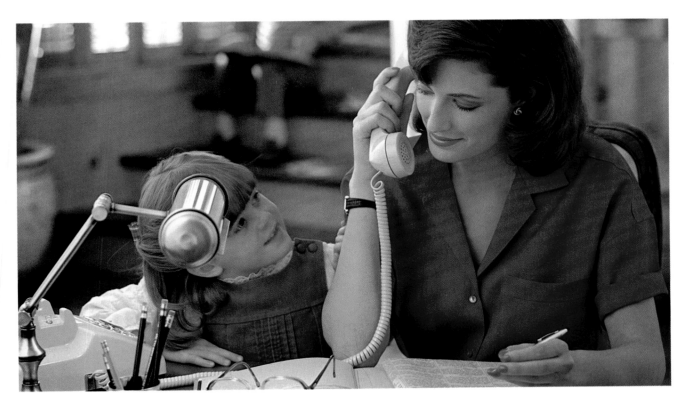

Gail's varied lifestyle calls for a beauty routine that's very versatile. By adapting her basic glamour makeup, she's able to achieve a range of looks to suit her many needs.

daytime and evening. Gail's normal-type hair has to be washed every two or three days. She always uses a conditioner to prevent tangling after shampooing; after every fourth shampoo, she uses an intensive conditioner for extra body and bounce.

To keep her *body* fit, Gail finds that she can work regular aerobic exercise into the afternoons she spends with her children by going bicycle riding with them. For relaxing stretches she attends an evening yoga class once or twice a week. The fragrances Gail favors express her sophisticated personality: for day she likes the softness of floral fragrances and for evening she prefers the gracious aura of aldehydics. She also has a wardrobe of fragrances to suit different occasions — herbaceous scents for sporty family outings, more sophisticated Orientals for daytime career meetings, and chypres for romantic evenings. Gail dresses her full figure for business days in clean, elongated lines in suit jackets, keeping her color scheme to dark, subtle hues. For evening she favors simple, elegant black, accented with dramatic accessories and large-scale jewelry. She looks for extended shoulders in many of her shirts and jackets to balance her full hips and legs, and wears long, straight-shaped skirts for dressy evenings.

Beauty musts: consistent skin and hair care emphasizing protection to maintain their normal condition; using contrasting colors to change her makeup look from day to evening; keeping wardrobe colors well coordinated, simple, and flattering; having a variety of fragrances to suit all her moods and occasions.

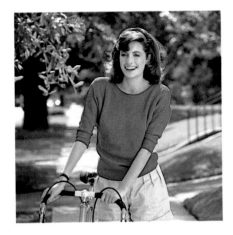

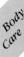

Body Care

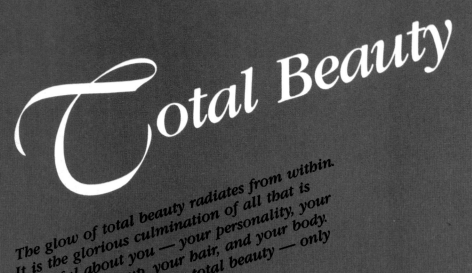

Total Beauty

The glow of total beauty radiates from within. It is the glorious culmination of all that is beautiful about you — your personality, your skin, your makeup, your hair, and your body. Only you hold the key to total beauty — only you can make the difference!

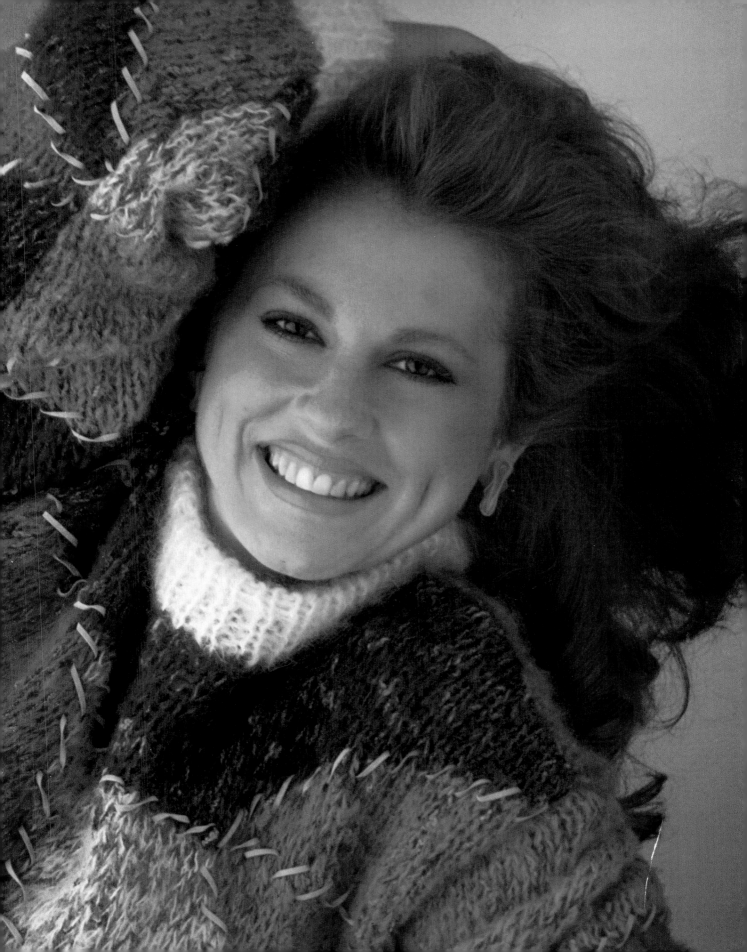

Making It Yours

You're a beautiful woman — you've worked hard at developing your own inner beauty, and we hope that all you've learned on the previous pages has helped to bring your own special beauty to the surface.

Your thoughtful answers to all the inventory questions throughout this book — especially on the following two pages — demonstrate your interest in every aspect of yourself. And because interest, caring, and commitment are the most important requirements for obtaining the best results from a complete beauty program, the effort, enthusiasm, and self-knowledge you invest in the guidelines you've learned will help make the difference.

But only you make the real difference — your time and effort, your special attention to details and problems, your caring about who you are and how you look. Making all of it yours — your inner beauty, your skin care, your glamorous makeup, your hair care, and your overall body care — means giving priority to your own health and beauty because you know how important they are to the way you feel about yourself and about the world around you. And you want to present your personal best, the most beautiful you possible, *every day* to *everyone*.

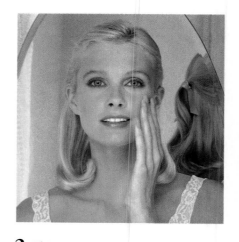

2 *Skin Care*
The basis of becoming and being your beautiful best; giving your skin the care and attention it needs by following the five steps to beautiful skin — cleanse, stimulate, freshen, moisturize, and protect; paying attention to the importance of your skin's health and appearance by really working at — and *enjoying* — the time and effort you devote to giving your skin a radiant glow, a smooth, even surface you can see, a soft, dewy texture you can feel: the perfect reflection of the very special way you've learned to care for yourself.

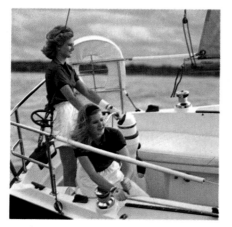

1 *Your Special Beauty*
Your understanding of who you are and your appreciation of your best inner qualities, wisely combined with those areas of your character you're always working on, always making better.

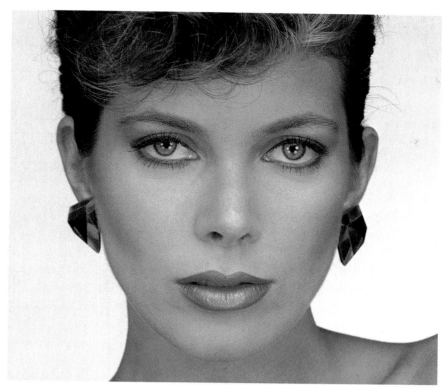

3 *Glamour Makeup*

The techniques and colors you choose to enhance your features — your eyes, lips, cheeks; the way you use the most sophisticated beauty knowledge to add a soft, natural glow to your face or to dramatize your looks with special effects; being adventurous and experimenting with makeup, learning new ways to look that you may never have thought were possible for you, understanding the nature of makeup and how to use it to your most beautiful advantage.

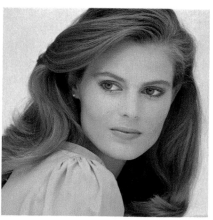

4 *Hair Care*

The special care you take to make the most of your hair's natural beauty: keeping it clean, soft, and conditioned, alive with shine and vitality, silky and lustrous, styled to enhance its natural characteristics and to frame your face beautifully.

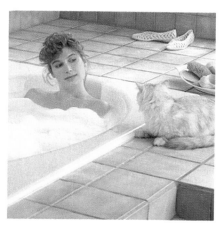

5 *Body Care*

The total image you project by putting it all together beautifully, paying attention to all the details — your hands, your feet, the sleep you get, and your fragrance choices and wardrobe — making them all part of a complete beauty routine that works for you, giving your body skin the extra care it needs to look soft and toned, to feel youthfully silken, and to retain its special beauty.

Taking a Final Look

Now that you have read *The Mary Kay Guide to Beauty,* take time to complete a few more statements and evaluate your overall appearance and feelings. Answer thoughtfully and honestly, and use your answers to help you set new goals for becoming all you can be.

This inventory includes a reference source of page numbers to give you extra instruction and inspiration in the specific areas covered in this book.

1. **I would like to increase my potential for inner beauty by concentrating more on the following areas:**
   - ☐ Self-confidence (*see pages 20 and 21*)
   - ☐ Intimacy (*see pages 22 and 23*)
   - ☐ Inner strength (*see pages 24 and 25*)
   - ☐ Versatility (*see pages 26 and 27*)
   - ☐ Direction (*see pages 28 and 29*)
   - ☐ Self-fulfillment (*see pages 30 and 31*)
   - ☐ Positive attitude (*see pages 32 and 33*)

2. **I understand the structure and composition of skin and the scientific basis for skin care.**
   - ☐ Yes
   - ☐ No (*see pages 40 to 43*)

3. **I would like my skin to look and feel (check all that apply):**
   - ☐ Clearer, with fewer clogged pores and breakouts (*see pages 56 to 59*)
   - ☐ Brighter and more translucent (*see pages 60 and 61*)
   - ☐ Fresher and better toned (*see pages 62 and 63*)
   - ☐ Softer, smoother, less dry, and better conditioned (*see pages 64 to 67*)
   - ☐ More youthful, more even toned in texture, and less wrinkled (*see pages 68 to 75*)

4. **I use a sunscreen to prevent sun damage on my facial skin:**
   - ☐ Whenever I will be outdoors, regardless of the season or the weather
   - ☐ Only when I know I will be directly exposed to the sun (*see pages 46, 47, and 69*)
   - ☐ Occasionally: when I go to the beach or boating (*see pages 46, 47, and 69*)
   - ☐ Infrequently: I like to get a tan (*see pages 46, 47, and 69*)

5. **I would like my face to appear (check either or both):**
   - ☐ More contoured and structured, with highlights (*see page 73*)
   - ☐ Less blotchy and irregular in coloring, with fewer obvious blemishes, lines, and dark areas (*see page 73*)

6. **I feel the time I currently spend on skin care is:**
   - ☐ Steadily improving the way my skin looks and feels
   - ☐ Not producing the results I'd like to see in my skin (*see pages 54 to 75*)

7. **I am happy with my total daytime makeup look:**
   - ☐ Always, or most of the time
   - ☐ Sometimes, but I need to learn new techniques (*see pages 82 to 111*)

8. **My makeup remains in good condition until I've used it up.**
   - ☐ Yes
   - ☐ No (*see page 83*)

9. **I need to improve my application of daytime (check all that apply):**
   - ☐ Cheek color (*see pages 88 to 91*)
   - ☐ Eyebrow pencil (*see pages 96 and 97*)
   - ☐ Eye shadow (*see pages 98 to 101*)
   - ☐ Eyeliner and/or eye-defining pencil (*see pages 102 and 103*)
   - ☐ Mascara (*see pages 104 and 105*)
   - ☐ Lip color (*see pages 108 and 109*)

10. **For special effects, I would like to learn how to experiment more with (check all that apply):**
   - ☐ My makeup colors (*see pages 84 to 87*)
   - ☐ Cheek contouring (*see pages 92 to 95*)
   - ☐ Enhancing the size, shape, and/or setting of my eyes (*see pages 106 and 107*)
   - ☐ Flattering eyeglass shapes (*see page 93*)
   - ☐ Enhancing the size and/or shape of my lips (*see pages 110 and 111*)

11. **I understand the structure and composition of hair and the scientific basis for hair care.**
☐ Yes
☐ No (*see pages 144 and 145*)

12. **I would like my hair to look and feel (check all that apply):**
☐ Cleaner and fresher (*see pages 150 and 151*)
☐ More flexible, shinier, less fly-away (*see pages 152 and 153*)
☐ Less damaged, with fewer split and broken ends (*see pages 154 and 155*)

13. **I am concerned about (check all that apply):**
☐ Dandruff (*see page 156*)
☐ Dry scalp (*see page 156*)
☐ Hair loss (*see pages 156 and 157*)
☐ How coloring and other treatments affect my hair (*see pages 158 and 159*)

14. **I need new hair styling ideas for (check all that apply):**
☐ Finding a hairstyle that suits the characteristics of my hair (*see pages 160 and 161*)
☐ Styling my hair to flatter my face (*see pages 162 to 165*)
☐ Adding versatility and special effects to my hairstyle (*see page 163*)

15. **I feel the time I currently spend on hair care is:**
☐ Steadily improving the way my hair looks and feels
☐ Not producing the results I'd like to see in my hair (*see pages 146 to 165*)

16. **I understand the structure and composition of body skin and the scientific basis for body skin care.**
☐ Yes
☐ No (*see pages 174 to 177*)

17. **I would like my body skin to look and feel (check all that apply):**
☐ Cleaner, fresher, and softer (*see pages 184 and 185*)
☐ Smoother; more polished looking; less rough on elbows, feet, and knees (*see pages 186 and 187*)
☐ Silkier, less dry (*see pages 188 and 189*)

18. **I use sunscreen on my body skin:**
☐ Whenever I am outdoors, regardless of the season or the weather
☐ Only when I know I will be directly exposed to the sun (*see pages 46, 47, 190, and 191*)
☐ Occasionally: when I go to the beach or boating (*see pages 46, 47, and 191*)
☐ Infrequently: I like to get a tan (*see pages 46, 47, and 191*)

19. **I need more information on the following areas of concern regarding body care (check all that apply):**
☐ My hands (*see pages 192 to 195*)
☐ My feet (*see pages 196 and 197*)
☐ Hair removal (*see pages 198 and 199*)
☐ During my pregnancy (*see pages 200 and 201*)

☐ Exercise (*see pages 202 and 203*)
☐ Sleep and relaxation (*see pages 204 to 207*)

20. **I'd like to learn new ideas about (check all that apply):**
☐ Fragrances that suit my individual personality, mood, and personal preferences (*see pages 210 and 211*)
☐ Buying the right fragrance for myself (*see pages 212 and 213*)
☐ Wearing fragrance in different ways (*see pages 212 and 213*)
☐ Using fragrance in layers (*see page 214*)

21. **I need new wardrobe and fashion tips (check all that apply):**
☐ To learn to shop more effectively for clothes (*see pages 216 and 217*)
☐ To flatter my figure type (*see pages 218 to 221*)

22. **Rank the following elements of your total beauty routine from one to five, beginning with the element that gives you the best results. Then reread the sections on those elements you feel still need some work.**
☐ Skin care (*see pages 38 to 77*)
☐ Daytime makeup (*see pages 78 to 113*)
☐ Special makeup effects (*see pages 114 to 141*)
☐ Hair care (*see pages 142 to 171*)
☐ Body care (*see pages 172 to 227*)

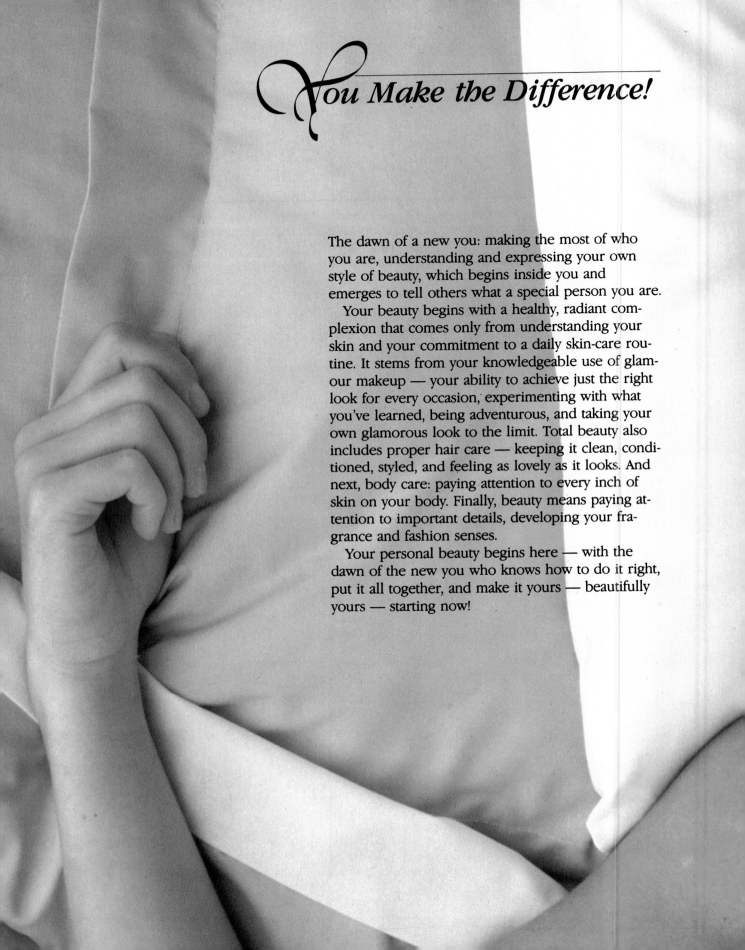

You Make the Difference!

The dawn of a new you: making the most of who you are, understanding and expressing your own style of beauty, which begins inside you and emerges to tell others what a special person you are.

Your beauty begins with a healthy, radiant complexion that comes only from understanding your skin and your commitment to a daily skin-care routine. It stems from your knowledgeable use of glamour makeup — your ability to achieve just the right look for every occasion, experimenting with what you've learned, being adventurous, and taking your own glamorous look to the limit. Total beauty also includes proper hair care — keeping it clean, conditioned, styled, and feeling as lovely as it looks. And next, body care: paying attention to every inch of skin on your body. Finally, beauty means paying attention to important details, developing your fragrance and fashion senses.

Your personal beauty begins here — with the dawn of the new you who knows how to do it right, put it all together, and make it yours — beautifully yours — starting now!

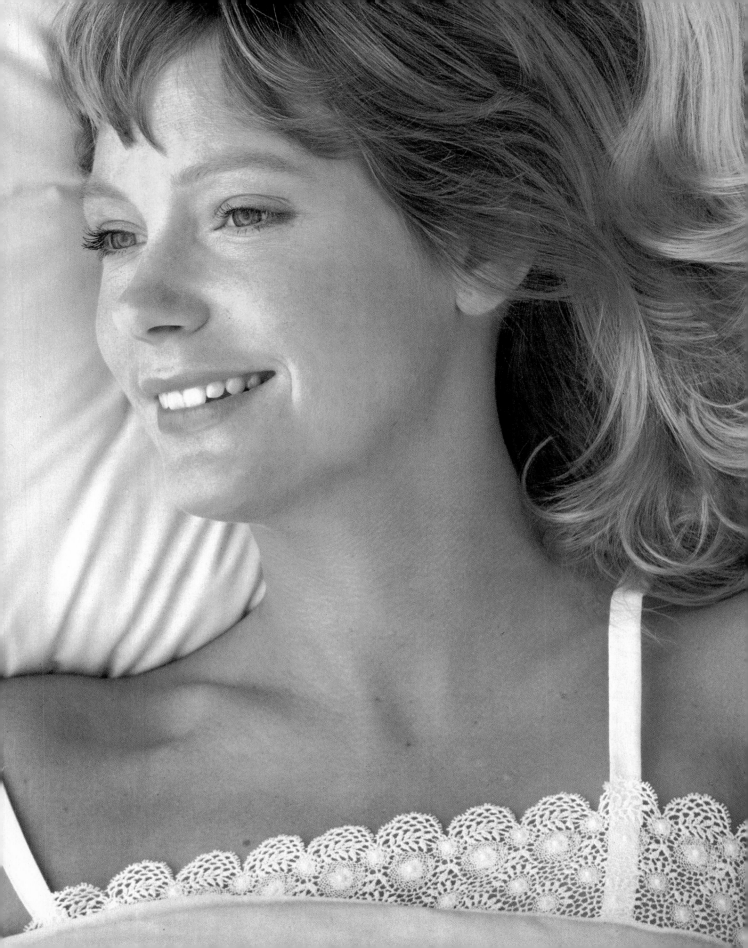

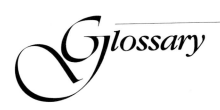

Glossary

Acid balance — the natural pH level of the skin's surface moisture; *see* pH

Aerobic exercise — activity that increases lung activity so that greater amounts of oxygen are absorbed and the heart rate is increased

Aldyhedics — one of five general fragrance categories

Alkali — any of various water-soluble mineral salts; a quality of detergent soaps

Allergen — a substance that produces an allergic reaction

Allergy — a hypersensitive reaction to environmental substances

Alopecia areata — a scalp disorder resulting in bald patches, believed to be related to "autoimmunity," or the body becoming allergic to its own chemicals

Androgen — a class of hormones that includes the male hormone testosterone; also, a component of some birth-control pills

Apocrine sweat glands — small tubes that secrete a milky substance that develops the characteristic human odor as it is decomposed by bacteria on the skin's surface; found mainly in the underarms, around the nipples, and in the groin

Arrector pili muscle — a muscle attached to each hair follicle that contracts as a result of cold or fear, making the hair shaft stand up straight and produce "goose bumps"

Astringent — causing the drawing together or constricting of tissue, such as skin or scalp; pore tightening; may also refer to a lotion that produces such action

Atopic dermatitis (*see* eczema)

Bacteria — one-celled organisms of various kinds, which often cause infection

Birthmark — dark areas on the skin produced by excessive pigmentation

Blood vessels — vessels that supply nutrients and oxygen to the skin; they help regulate body temperature by contracting and expanding in response to external stimuli

Browbone — the usually prominent area just under the outer half of the eyebrow; a ridgelike bone found under the length of the eyebrow

Callus — hard, tough skin created by friction

Capillaries — minute blood vessels that connect arteries and veins

Chloasma — "mask of pregnancy," dark patches on cheeks, near mouth or brow, associated with hormonal changes of pregnancy

Chypres — one of five general fragrance categories

Collagen — a protein substance found in connective or supportive tissue such as the dermis

Comedo — technical name for skin lesions, which include blackheads (open comedones) and whiteheads (closed comedones)

Comedogenic — causing comedones — whiteheads or blackheads

Contouring (as related to makeup) — adding dimension with shadows and highlights to any of the facial features

Cortex (hair) — the center part or layer surrounding the innermost layer, called the medulla, of the hair shaft, just inside the cuticle, or external layer of hair

Cosmetic — a beautifying agent, usually for the face or body

Cuticle (hair) — the thin, hard outer surface of the hair shaft; covers the cortex

Cuticle (nails) — the hard skin at the base and sides of fingernails and toenails

Definition (as related to makeup) — emphasis or accent on the shape or contour of any of the facial features

Dehydration — the loss or absence of moisture or water

Demarcation (in makeup application) — the obvious boundary line between two shades or textures; the unappealing effect of makeup that is not well blended and/or shows an unattractive line between skin and makeup

Depilatory — a chemical compound for removing hair

Dermatology — the medical study and science of the structure, function, and diseases of the skin

Dermis — the fibrous skin layer beneath the epidermis, composed primarily of elastin and collagen

Detergent — a cleansing substance that allows oil and water to combine

DNA — *d*eoxyribo*n*ucleic *a*cid, a complex chromosomal component of the nuclei, or centers, of living cells, which determine individual hereditary characteristics

Dormancy — a period of rest, when growth ceases (in hair, for example)

Eccrine sweat glands — small coiled tubes that open up on the skin's surface as pores, bringing water and waste products (perspiration) to the skin's surface

Eczema — a wide range of skin problems, usually related to an extreme susceptibility to some form of irritation or allergies

Elasticity — the capacity (as of skin or hair) to stretch without losing shape

Elastin — a substance that forms a principal component of elastic fiber or tissue in the body, found in the dermis layer; it keeps the skin supple

Emery board — a cardboard nail-filing implement coated with a fine-grained aluminum oxide or other abrasive mineral; used to grind and polish the nail gently

Emollient — a substance that softens and soothes, usually by depositing oil on the skin's surface

Epidermis — the outermost layer of skin cells covering the body; the skin we can see

Fibrocytes — cells that produce high-tensile-strength fibers made of the protein collagen, the "structural steel" of the skin

Hair follicles — tubes in which hair grows; they originate in the dermis and extend upward through the epidermis, forming the surrounding tissue for growing hair

Heredity — the genetic transmission of characteristics from parents to offspring.

Hormones — substances produced by several of the body's organs that stimulate other organs to function by chemical activity

Horny layer (*see* **stratum corneum**)

Hydrate — to moisturize or add water

Hyperactivity — a high level of activity in the functioning of organs or glands (such as sebaceous glands)

Humectants — water-attracting, or moisture-binding, substances

Humidity — the amount of moisture or water held in the atmosphere

Iris (of the eye) — the colored circular area surrounding the eye's pupil

Irritant — any condition or substance that produces irritation

Keratin — a tough, fibrous protein that is part of the outer layer of the skin's epidermis and of the hair and fingernails

Lubrication — the coating on a material or skin which promotes mobility and reduces friction

Manicure stick — a nail-care implement made of soft wood (like orange), usually with a pointed end for cleaning and a flat, round end for grooming the nail cuticle

Matte finish — an even-toned, nonshiny surface quality (as of skin to which translucent powder has been applied)

Medulla (hair) — the innermost, softest substance that forms the center of some hair shafts

Melanin — a dark skin and hair pigment

Melanocytes — cells producing melanin

Mid-shaft split — the unraveling of the ropelike fibers of the cortex in the middle of a shaft of hair

Natural bristle brush — a brush made from natural animal hair (often boar) rather than synthetics such as plastic; generally considered to be gentler on the hair and scalp

Opaque — not allowing light to penetrate — the opposite of transparent; dense coverage

Oxidation — the combination of any substance with oxygen

Palette (of makeup) — an array of several different colors packaged conveniently in a single container

Papule — a small, inflamed elevation of the skin

Patina — a fine, smooth film, usually glowing, that forms on a surface

pH (*potential of Hydrogen*) — a measure of acidity or alkalinity of a solution or substance; 7 is neutral pH; lower pH numbers represent acid pH, high pH numbers indicate alkaline pH; the natural pH of skin is slightly acidic, or below 7 pH

Pigment — any coloring agent, such as melanin, in the skin and hair

Pollutant — impure or unclean contaminating materials

Psoriasis — a skin condition characterized by patches of scaly, shedding skin; most often develops on the scalp, knees, and elbows

Pumice — a porous, lightweight, abrasive volcanic stone used to soften and polish hard, tough, or callused skin

Regenerate — re-create living material, or renew functioning

Rosacea — a face rash that produces redness and pimples in adults, especially on the nose, mid-forehead, chin, and cheeks

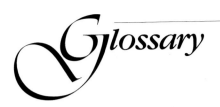

Glossary

Saturated color — dense, opaque makeup colors, applied so that little of the natural skin tones show through

Scar — connective tissue visible at the skin's surface that fills in the opening of a cut

Sebaceous glands — oil-producing glands attached to hair follicles

Seborrheic dermatitis — a common skin disorder that produces scaling and itching of the facial skin; may be associated with excessive secretion of sebum

Sebum — a semiliquid oil secreted by the sebaceous glands that lubricate the skin's surface

Shafts (of hair) — individual strands of hair

Sloughing — the shedding of an outer layer of dead tissue from a living structure, such as skin

SPF (Sun Protection Factor) — the numerical rating on sunscreens that indicates the level of protection they can provide the skin from ultraviolet radiation; the higher the SPF number, the greater a sunscreen's protective capacity

Split end — the unraveling of the ropelike fibers of the cortex at the end of a shaft of hair

Stratum corneum — the flat, dead skin cells that form a protective outer layer on the surface of the skin; also called horny layer

Subcutaneous — below the skin

Sunscreen — a preparation that blocks the harmful burning rays of the sun

Translucent — allowing some light to penetrate or pass through, without being completely transparent

T-zone — the T-shaped area of the face formed by the forehead, the nose, and the chin, which sometimes tends to be oiler than other facial areas

Ultraviolet — the range of light wavelengths (usually from the sun) between violet radiation in the visible spectrum and the invisible x-ray spectrum; such rays are harmful to the skin

Vitiligo — light patches on the skin resulting from the lack of melanin in a specific area

Water-resistant — repelling moisture or water; not easily rinsed away by water

Water-soluble — the quality of dissolving in water; easily removed with water

Mary Kay Cosmetics, Inc., fully supports skin-care education and research through: Harvard University–the Massachusetts Institute of Technology, Division of Health Sciences and Technology; the University of Texas Health Science Center at Dallas; and the "Skin Deep" exhibit, developed by Mary Kay Cosmetics, Inc., in cooperation with the American Academy of Dermatology, the Dermatology Foundation, the Chicago Dermatology Society, and the Museum of Science and Industry in Chicago, Illinois.

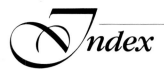

Index

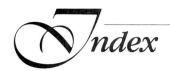
All photographs in *The Mary Kay Guide to Beauty* are the work of Photographers, Inc., with the exception of the following: 7, Francesco Scavullo; **13 and 25**, Ilse Thoma/The Image Bank; **14 (top) and 56**, Hank Londoner/The Image Bank; **14 (bottom) and 46 (bottom)**, Miguel/The Image Bank; **15**, Nancy Brown/The Image Bank; **16 (top)**, **29, 32, 33, 34 (top)**, **42, and 204**, Skip Hine; **16 (bottom)**, D. Kugelmeier/The Image Bank; **17**, John Stember/The Image Bank; **18**, Philip M. Prosen/The Image Bank; **19 (top)**, Whitney Lane/The Image Bank; **19 (bottom)**, Richard Steedman/The Image Bank; **20**, Elisabeth Weiland/Photo Researchers; **21 (top)**, Steve Niedorf/The Image Bank; **21 (bottom) and 201**, Elyse Lewin/The Image Bank; **22**, Werner Bokelberg/The Image Bank; **23**, George Hausman/The Image Bank; **24**, Jay Maisel/The Image Bank; **26**, Paulo Rocha/The Image Bank; **27**, Alvis Upitis/The Image Bank; **28**, Steve Dunnell/The Image Bank; **30**, Edward Leptau/Photo Researchers; **31**, Faustino R/The Image Bank; **34 (bottom)**, Bard Martin/The Image Bank; **35**, Jack Ward/The Image Bank; **43 (right)**, **180, and 205**, Larry Dale Gordon/The Image Bank; **45**, Rosemary Howard; **46 (top)**, Susan McCartney/Photo Researchers; **68**, Jean Louis Sauverzac/The Image Bank; **80**, Janeart, LTD/The Image Bank; **81 (left)**, Gabe Palmer/The Image Bank; **81 (right)**, Brett H. Froomer/The Image Bank; **105 (lower right)**, Michael Salas/The Image Bank; **191 (top)**, John Kelly/The Image Bank; **191 (bottom)**, David Brownell/The Image Bank.